I Want to Make You Smile

I Want to Make You Smile

A family memoir of resilence in the age of Alzheimer's

Lindelwa Ntutela

Warrior Princess Nation, LLC

Warrior Publishing, a division of
Warrior Princess Nation, LLC
6935 Aliante Pkwy Ste 104 #423
North Las Vegas, NV 89084
for information email info@warriorprincessnation.com

First Printing, 2025

Table of Contents

Dedication

To my beloved sister, Smileth Ncunyiswa, whose enduring smile and warrior spirit have illuminated my path. Your journey through Alzheimer's has profoundly altered my life's trajectory.

To the unwavering dedication of Smileth's caregivers, home health aides, physiotherapists, and visiting wound specialists whose compassion and tireless devotion have provided immeasurable support and care.

To my sister, Pam (aka 'Posh'), may I inherit even half of your strength.

Foreword

Alzheimer's disease is a journey that countless individuals and families embark on every year, navigating uncharted territories of memory loss, cognitive decline, and emotional resilience. As we continue to unravel the complexities of this debilitating condition, it becomes increasingly clear that awareness, education, and compassion are our most potent tools in the fight against Alzheimer's.

This book offers hope, guidance, and support for those affected by Alzheimer's. Through Lindelwa's research on the condition, personal experiences, and stories of resilience, we gain a deeper understanding of the disease and its far-reaching impact. From the intricacies of diagnosis and treatment to the emotional nuances of caregiving and coping, this book tackles the complexities of Alzheimer's with sensitivity, clarity, and empathy. She demystifies the myths, especially in the African communities, associated with Alzheimer's. One of these myths is that Alzheimer's affects people who do not actively engage their minds. As mentioned in the book, Smileth was a principal of a top-performing high school in Soweto. She was one of the best English teachers. Her dedication to education and her passion for empowering young minds inspired countless lives.

With Alzheimer's dementia rates steadily increasing in our diverse communities across all provinces, the need for culturally sensitive support and practical caregiving solutions has become critical. I Want to Make You Smile is more than just a personal story for the Ntutela family– it's a testament to the strength and courage of caregivers and care recipients everywhere, particularly those from marginalized communities who often face unique challenges in accessing support and resources. May their story inspire you, comfort you, and remind you that you are not alone.

As we strive for greater awareness, improved care, and, ultimately, a cure for Alzheimer's, this memoir serves as a powerful reminder of the human spirit's capacity for love, adaptability, and perseverance. May it spark a deeper conversation about the complexities of Alzheimer's, the importance of community-based care, and the need for greater support and understanding for those affected by this disease.

This book is a lighthouse of hope and understanding, offering universal lessons on resilience and the power of family bonds. It is a must-read for anyone touched by dementia, those interested in cultural narratives, and readers seeking stories of emotional depth and human connection in the age of Alzheimer's. May the stories, insights, and expertise shared within these pages inspire, educate, and comfort all those touched by Alzheimer's, and may we continue to move forward together, fueled by hope, compassion, and determination.

Dr. Mfezo Blossom 'Blondie' Mokgata, MD
Medical Certification Panel
Morningside Manor, Sandton
Johannesburg, South Africa

Preface

"You Will Remember For Me."

I take inspiration for this book from two related words: 'parach' and 'telos.' In Hebrew, the word 'parach' signifies sprout and blossom. "Sprout" describes when a flower breaks out or blooms, emitting a sweet fragrance into the air. When I read my Parach Daily Devotionals each morning, I am both commanding a closed flower to open and being commanded, in this season, to open up my spirit, blossom, and sprout. The Greek word 'telos' which means deeper purpose, held great significance for framing the narrative for this work.

In 2022, I had a dream in which a strong, invisible force pushed me off the edge of a cliff. In this dream, I was eager to discern whether the individuals pushing me were friends or foes. I felt the weight of their presence as they stood behind me, their hands on my back, conversing casually yet goading me to jump. There was no aura of hate. "Go on, take a step forward," a man's voice instructed, and I hesitated. With gentle, non-coercive pushes, I was jostled forward. I wasn't fearful but more concerned about the identity behind the voice instructing me to leap.

As the pushing hands ceased their resistance, I broke free and stepped forward on my own accord. The descent from the cliff was steep, with the cliff towering as high as a skyscraper in New York or Dubai. Yet, I soared above these skyscrapers with inexplicable ease, my arms outstretched like the wings of a majestic bird. I couldn't locate my landing spot; the distance I would travel before hitting the ground was obscured by fog. Leaving the cliff behind, I soared through the thick, cloud-like mist, passing buildings and beginning my descent into a vast, open space illuminated by the break of day. Suddenly, I found myself floating on a parachute as if my body were strapped onto a flying railroad with metal wings attached to my back and lower torso. I could hear the sound of metal rails neatly adjusting themselves, protecting me and preparing me for a precise landing. A metal helmet secured onto my head, and I glided through the atmosphere, past hills, towering structures, bridges, rivers, trees, and multi-unit residences.

Drawing closer to the ground at the speed of a fast-moving rocket, I glimpsed a fluffy white cloud forming beneath my feet above a cool, grassy surface sprinkled with tiny droplets of water. As I landed, the soft cloud cushioned my descent without any physical impact. Walking away from the direction of the cliff into my waking consciousness, I pondered the reason behind being pushed off that cliff and who initiated it. Wait! All that preparation with state-of-the-art wings, rail glides, and helmets, and I'm here on this soft earth without the anticipated drama? I'm now walking on dewy green grass unscathed, stepping onto a bushy path toward a new, unfamiliar horizon with the boldness, focus, and clarity of an eagle. How?

I conquered my long-standing fears when I stepped forward and took a leap off of that cliff. It was a moment of deliverance that trumped every experience of crash-and-burn, defeat, delay, backsliding, and entrapment I had become familiar with, freeing my spirit to fly high.

I have had many prophetic dreams in my adult life. Eleven years into my sister Ncuncu's onset Alzheimer's dementia diagnosis, it dawned on me that my dream was preparing me for a new role. It was a revelation of her repetitive request to me when she was still able to talk. "You will remember for me, Dzedze," she would say. The request was a reiterated echo that kept me awake most nights. This was not a request to help her remember people's faces and names when she could no longer remember them. Her insistence that I remember for her was a call that appealed to me to take action. This was my assigned role, to honor my sister concretely.

In the spirit realm, I was being assigned as the family sledgehammer to break down walls, concrete, intractable obstacles of tradition, old grudges, and festering family secrets, and find inner strength to battle with and defeat challenges along the way. Diving into my sister's experiences with a shocking brain disease, I was tasked to remember for her, articulate her struggle, and document her resilient spirit to fight against cognitive decline. This would be no easy feat; I would have to walk with others on this journey. Since I had moved from New York City to California, my journal had become my refuge. In my daily entries, I had taken the time to log an emotion or mood and the choices I had to make in the face of a family crisis. This was also not a moment to reflect on broad, existential questions about spirituality, identity, or mortality that resonate universally. In my ruminations, I became drawn more to the human experience, real-life, everyday joys and sorrows that bind us together, challenging us to recognize our shared humanity, and questions placing my mother's child's encounter with a monster disease at the center of discourse and conversation about that disease. My sister's journey drew me into that deeper purpose. I wanted to know what makes a beautiful life, a meaningful life and how we might honor the lives and wishes of those whose care is in our hands when they can no longer speak for themselves. To do this, I would have to flesh out the nexus of our collective life story as the three remaining siblings in our nuclear family, women connected by a shared generation, biology, loss, and grief. Throughout the writing process, Ncuncu was a constant presence, before and after she lost her speech. In my writing, her presence and active participation illuminated our collective struggles and triumphs as a family, and I wanted her story to become a lens through which readers could view their own lives and frailties.

Our sister's story puts a face to a misunderstood disease in a South African context. Sharing our family's personal and collective caregiving experiences, her story holds a mirror to shed a reflective light on Alzheimer's disease as a growing African and global concern. And so, as I sat by my sister's bedside, feeding her a bowl of oatmeal, remembering events, tracking the trajectory and contours of this disease from 2012, scribbling journal notes, analyzing videos and photographs, and watching her memories gradually slip away like grains of sand, I knew I had to document our experiences reflexively in a memoir. Ncuncu's struggle with Alzheimer's dementia became my driving force, and her resilience was the lifeblood - a telos breathed into every word, and total surrender to the divine Spirit to guide me into all truth and teach me all things.

I

Beneath the Palm Tree

In the heart of Kelvin, a suburb in Johannesburg where the sun blazes and memories cling like dust, a palm tree with a firm, spiky trunk stands in the corner of a small front yard garden. Its crown reaches for the sky, and its leaves sway amid green shrubbery, whispering secrets to the wind. Beneath its shelter, a retired African female teacher sits and finds solace. The palm tree, roots digging deep, seeking nourishment in barren suburban soil, has seen her prepare lesson plans for numerous upcoming weeks' classes and witnessed her dreams, joys, silent fears, and anxieties. On a black, patio glass table an old, chipped, pink fruit bowl she inherited from her mother holds memories of shared stories. She traces the contours of the brim with her left hand and stops to remember something. Yes, she has kept this fruit bowl for many years. As it chips on the glass edges, so does her recollection.

Born in Emgwali, a lush, picturesque village in Stutterheim, a school district where our mother worked, the teacher grew up in Mhlahlane, our ancestral village in a small rural town known as Tsomo. She came to live in this Jo'burg city as a girl when apartheid's iron grip shaped her childhood and choked her and her mother's dreams. Settling down in Dube Village, Mofolo, and Protea North, these townships provided the fertile ground that shaped her prolific teaching, sharpened her educational leadership skills, and provided all the ingredients she needed to succeed. She taught high school in a Johannesburg radius, and much like the palm tree in her front yard, it is in this same community that she emerged from the soil like a resilient seed, determined to thrive despite the harsh South African landscape.

This is the story of Ncuncu, a sharp-witted, take-charge kind of woman who moved up the ranks to school principal in Soweto. She knew she could subvert the structures of tribalism, and ethnic favoritism that undermined her mother, a school teacher who could not be promoted to a higher level because she was Xhosa. Education for her was a premium, not just essential, but also something to be treasured and invested in. The daughter of two elementary school teachers, she completed her Junior Secondary Teacher's Certificate at Lovedale Teachers College in Alice, Eastern Cape, and studied part-time for her Bachelor's and Master's degrees in Education, preparing to engage a new generation of students with a transformational pedagogy. Her son, now married with four children, grew into young adulthood at private preparatory schools, and his mother was relentless in enrolling him at the City University of New York, where I worked as a faculty member. But then, in 2012, she was diagnosed with Alzheimer's, a progressive, neurodegenerative disease, the onset of which often gets mistaken for normal aging.

Doctors pointed out a faulty depth perception. Ncuncu missed the stairs, tripped, and fell very easily. She lost direction driving home many times. Once, she missed her normal off-ramp from the freeway and pulled over into a gas station. There, she asked a stranger if he could ride with her and help her navigate home safely. That defining moment forced her into retirement against her will. She had to cope not only with the burden of knowledge about gradual cognitive decline but also accept that she was also leaving behind a profession she had come to love, one that sustained and defined for her the meaning of life itself.

This is also the story of our family, bound by blood and burdened by the weight of disenfranchised grief and trauma. At its heart lies our sister's journey, a struggle with memory loss. Our collective family battle serves as a poignant backdrop to the complexities of our shared history. In the maze of our family's narrative, grief, loss, and resilience have intertwined, weaving a complex mosaic. Through our shared experiences, we confront the ghosts of the past, bearing witness to the silent struggles that shape our present reality. As we journey forward together through the depths of Alzheimer's dementia, we carry with us the echoes of those who came before us. Their stories are etched into the very fabric of our being, a testament to the enduring power of memory, love, empathy, and family resilience.

Grief weaves its way in and out of our lives, all of us. It is a tapestry of emotions that bind us to the memories of those we hold dear. Yet, not all grief is openly acknowledged, socially accepted, or publicly mourned. In the shadowy corners of our existence lie the silent whispers of profound sorrow that result from non-death losses, defying the boundaries of traditional mourning rituals. For those grappling with the relentless progression of Alzheimer's disease, grief can cast a long shadow, its tendrils reaching deep into the recesses of the soul. It mimics what has been termed stigmatized loss that accompanies diagnoses like AIDS, mental ill-health, and chronic substance-related issues. These losses are characterized by stigma that can occur at interpersonal, intrapersonal, and structural levels as a result of labeling, stereotypes, social separation, and discrimination.

The idea that individuals with Alzheimer's dementia become "different people" or "strangers" is a common misconception. As close kin, it is said, we "lose" our loved ones to Alzheimer's dementia, and they become unrecognizable or fundamentally different. However, research and experts in the field emphasize that this is not true. Inside, the person remains the same individual they were before the onset of Alzheimer's. Their core personality, emotions, and memories persist, even if their cognitive abilities decline. Providing direct care for Ncuncu at home has allowed us to dispel this notion. We have missed the witty, quirky, critical-thinking arguments and thought-provoking conversations we shared with our feisty sibling. But we have never lost our sister, and despite the ravages of the disease, she has not become a 'stranger.' Inside, she has always been there. Her essence never changed, and she never morphed into a different person from the sibling we have always known. As family caregivers, our experiences with her have mostly converged, differing in nuance brought about by our individual interaction and engagement with her.

As an ethnographic, action researcher, I have been able to hone and refine the skill of participant engagement. I live and work in a country thousands of miles away and am only able to visit home once a year and twice if I have saved enough money to afford travel. On each visit, I have interacted with my sister, verbally and nonverbally, and tracked and compiled notes, photographs, and video footage changes that I observed. In the last few years, I discovered an invaluable communication style through which I could understand where she was with the disease daily. Each visit, irrespective of the stage of the disease, takes only a few days for my sister to recognize me, but she does not forget me. I watch and notice her great effort to remember the new voice, my voice, amid familiar caregivers around her. "Dzedze!" she will call out when memory and recognition return. We whisper in conversation in the middle of the night, and together, we giggle like we did in the twin bed we shared as young girls in Soweto. Like we did before the diagnosis. I cannot bear to watch her forehead wrinkle up, and her eyelids blink faster when she senses that I am leaving for the airport again.

This book debunks the myth that Alzheimer's turns loved ones into strangers, showing instead that while cognitive decline happens, the essence of the person remains intact. We emphasize the importance of empathetic communication in providing effective caregiving for individuals with Alzheimer's dementia. It is crucial to allow the person with the condition to steer conversations, responding to her chosen subjects. Often, for Ncuncu, conversations involve school kids or school events. Where her memories seem to be caught up in the period when she was a school teacher or school principal, we shift and change the subject on hand, and join in her topic of interest at that given moment. We have come to know that Alzheimer's is a complex disease that attacks cognition, behavior, and communication abilities. When Ncuncu speaks, we listen and learn from her. Earlier in the diagnosis, and until she could no longer express herself verbally, we learned to listen and learn even from the divergent thinking that derailed her from one idea to the next. We suspended our opinions or judgments and trained other caregivers to do the same. With an exploration of our individual or team communication with her throughout all the stages of the disease, we share strategies that help facilitate interaction even in advanced stages. We believe the best communication style is to avoid contradicting the person living with the disease. It may be difficult to give up the upper hand if you are a caregiver driven by the need for control. However, it is advised that caregivers avoid a "me versus her" approach but rather listen to the person with dementia and learn from them.

Each patient's journey with Alzheimer's is unique, and they progress through the stages of the disease differently. In the thick of our sister's cognitive anguish, we have discovered that her smile is a way of speaking when there are no more words to say. With it, she conveys her feelings, emotions, and unspoken words. As it was in her active life, music and random, unchoreographed dance moves were the most explicit expressions of her inner core. They embodied the family and social life she greatly cherished. She danced with her smile and deeply connected with whoever watched her dance as if to say, "Look at me, I can make you smile." You couldn't help but respond with a giggle or a whoop and a holler. She could be seen in the pews of Bethesda Methodist, her home church, or at an event at the Central Methodist Church in the city, singing and thumping her Bible to her favorite Hymn 116, "Lizalis'idinga lakho," and good rhythm was sure to accompany the song with a sway of hips and a knowing smile. Hers was more than a smile. With it, she was saying more than you could decipher. It was an invitation for you to hear the music in her dance moves. It was the music that danced, and she was only a vessel for you to hear it.

In Ncuncu's story, we capture some of the songs she loved that stood out from very different cultural settings. If she sang Handel's "And the glory, the glory of the Lord," she would stop in the middle of the room and emphatically exclaim, "Shall be-e-e-e revealed" with her head tilted back, eyes looking up, and palms of her hands open high and wide in a posture of divine praise. We simply let these songs dance, and we follow their rhythm. It stops the pain for a while and heals our own emotions, releasing strong feelings and more memories of Ncuncu's life trajectory. Singing, smiling, and performing to herself and others became a key symbolic element of her survival and resilience in the face of a devastating disease. Then, gradually, walking, singing, and dancing came to an end; language itself stopped, and she was confined to a wheelchair. Yet despite the challenges she faced, her enduring smile continued to serve as a symbol of resilience and inner strength. With her eyes now closed, facial skin tightly compressed, and her arms unable to lift high in a posture of praise and worship, she smiles with sorrowful intensity, and we know intuitively that Handel's Messiah is not lost to her memory. Through Ncuncu's story, we have witnessed the gradual erosion of physical strength, fading echoes of memory, and the silent lament of unspoken truths, each stage in the progression a testament to the enduring power of human agency.

Chapter II introduces readers to Ncuncu's world before the diagnosis and highlights a sibling love that had always been present, ensuring physical and emotional security and support in the context of a family headed by our married but husbandless mother. The chapter describes a rootedness in the intersecting systems of racial segregation and patriarchy, where our family dynamics were characterized by male domination in a pseudo-polygamous formation. This setting shaped Ncuncu's personality, her relationships with family, her dreams, and hopes, formed the backdrop for her professional work, and foreshadowed signs that something might be wrong.

In Chapter III, a diagnosis is announced, and we confront the initial reactions of Ncuncu and her family to it. This chapter highlights the disbelief, fear, and grief that accompany the realization of what lies ahead. We follow Ncuncu's journey as she adapts and adjusts her life, to prepare for gradual loss of memory, identity, and sense of self.

Chapter IV, Posh's Home-Based Care, is an informative account of Posh's remarkable role as a staunch pillar in caring for Ncuncu in her own home. In the case of our beloved sister, it became imperative to shield her from the sting of stigma. Thus, we made a solemn vow to ensure she remained in the warmth of her home, regardless of the sacrifices required. In this chapter, Posh resigns from her job in the Northwest and begins a support and caring system that defies the need for nursing homes, but it is not without challenges. This chapter bears witness to both the fragility of our sister's existence and captures the depth of Posh's commitment and the spiritual dimension of her role as caregiver.

Chapter V curates a constellation of memories, a cluster of surprising moments, ad-lib sayings, and random actions that reveal that Ncuncu has a lesson for us to learn. In the advanced stage of Alzheimer's dementia, she demonstrates a certain intuitive awareness that enables her not only to cope in the face of adversity but also to adapt and maintain cognitive function beyond what might be expected based solely on memory-related factors. The essence of resilience here is the mental and emotional strength that goes beyond mere memory function and that allows her to navigate the challenges posed by the disease. This chapter underscores the importance of understanding and supporting the resilience of Alzheimer's patients as a crucial aspect of living with a challenging and intractable cognitive health condition.

In Chapter VI, Destigmatizing and Humanizing Alzheimer's Disease, we engage in a discussion about the impact of stigma associated with the condition. Stigmatization related to Alzheimer's disease can manifest in various ways, perpetuating misconceptions and negatively impacting affected individuals and their families. In this chapter, we offer a social justice lens, a perspective that helps examine the challenges of Alzheimer's disease beyond individual circumstances. This way of seeing encourages us to consider broader social, political, economic, and cultural factors when addressing various challenges. Thus, the chapter is also a call to action for families in Africa and its diaspora who have members living with Alzheimer's disease to consider ways to effectively manage their loved one's symptoms and their self-care by framing Alzheimer's discussions through a social justice lens to dispel myths, promote equity, and humanize the experiences of those affected.

Finally, Chapter VII highlights the transformative power of pain and emphasizes how caregivers find purpose amidst difficulties. Just as a stone must break for the heart of a fruit to stand in the sun, caregivers often experience emotional pain. In this chapter, we discuss the sacrifices they make, the emotional toll, and the moments when their understanding deepens. We explore how pain, derived from self-chosen sacrifice, can lead to growth, compassion, and a more profound connection with loved ones and the healing power of empathy.

II

Rooted in the Colluding Systems of Apartheid and Patriarchy

She was named Smileth at birth and lived up to her name right away. Mother said she was born smiling, and she was a very cheerful, round-faced little girl who brought happiness throughout the family and village. All children on my mother's side of the family were given names that assigned certain gender expectations to them. A person's name implicates other people's lives and impacts family unity and interconnectedness. It has meaning for the greater good and greater whole; it becomes a microcosm of collective consciousness and responsibility. Our mother's name, Boniswa, "the one gifted with second sight," cast her in the role of family visionary. Across the aisle, not so much. Birth names did not have to follow a defined pattern with concise gender expectations.

Our father, the family patriarch, was named Ntsikana—a name evoking the central pillar that holds the roof of a house together, preventing it from collapsing. Some family members believed he was named after the great Xhosa intellectual and prophet Ntsikana, who pioneered a radical form of Christianity. This visionary faith subverted Western Christianity, refusing to let it dominate African spirituality, and left an enduring legacy on Black consciousness. Yet, this interpretation of his name never truly took hold. Our father was a very good singer and, occasionally, filled in as a preacher at our church in Mhlahlane, but soon became distracted by the things of the world. His brother was named Dumentlango—the one who would roar from afar across the desert.

For a time, my parents' names seemed to suggest a union destined for greatness, a match made in heaven. But eventually, the pillar could not hold, and things fell apart. Perhaps it was just as well that the prophetic version of his name never gained much popularity.

Ncuncu followed Posh in the birth order, and her name signified a catharsis that would restore joy and laughter to a family that was rapidly becoming dysfunctional. They nicknamed me Dzedze, because, as they stated, I evolved differently. I didn't crawl as a baby but jumped like a flea from the sitting position to wherever I needed to be. When I finally walked, I was so bow-legged that I waddled from side to side like a 'drunken master,' so my family switched between Dzedze and "Gxadada," and it lasted a lifetime. For each one of us, a role is enshrined in our names. As Lindelwa, I arrived as a joyfully anticipated baby. Beyond being the third in a line of siblings, my mother held higher expectations for me. I was the missing puzzle piece entrusted with adding value to our family. Without my arrival, completeness would remain elusive.

Ncuncu's English name translated into Ncunyiswa, which, in isiXhosa means 'the one born with a smile,' also, 'the one who makes us smile.' Our mother spoiled her as a toddler by singing a special, affectionate song popular in her generation. It was called "My bonnie lass, she smileth," a song attributed to Thomas Morley, a prominent English composer. In Scottish language, the word 'bonnie' means "pretty." Whenever the song played on the radio, Ncuncu would immediately stop and smile because she knew it was about her. It called her name. The song portrays a scene where the speaker admires the smile of his beloved, finding joy and beauty in it. Ncuncu knew how to smile like a bonnie lass, a beautiful, endearing young girl. She walked in brisk short steps and grew up to become a sassy 5'2" woman. Her name, Smileth, reflects her disposition and character as a cheerful and joyful person, much like the subject of Morley's song.

As a growing girl-child, the late 1950s were a period marked by relative quietude in the political climate of South Africa. Ncuncu lived largely in the comfort and protection of the countryside in the beautiful rural village of Stutterheim where our mother was a grade school teacher. In Mhlahlane, our paternal village, our parents' house was only a few yards from our grandmother's, allowing for easy access and communal childcare amongst the many women of my family who included my mother, grandmother, other mothers, father's sisters, and uncle's wives.

Ncuncu, Posh, and I developed a close relationship. We were raised by our grandmother, Letisha, a strict but compassionate Christian woman who, as a product of the Royal Readers, spoke perfect English – the Queen's language. Ncuncu was her favorite, and a child loved throughout the village. Grandma protected us and met all our basic needs in our childhood while our mother was away working in Johannesburg, and our father lived with other women and started new families with them.

One of my fondest memories is when we played on a rocky strip of land between our house and Auntie Nancy's, our neighbor. We often walked as far as emthonjeni, a tiny well of fresh, clean water jutting out of the ground where white geese fed and rested. One day, the geese noticed Ncuncu, as they often did when she was in their presence. It was December, Mama was visiting from the city, and she had decorated Red House, our childhood home, with beautiful, shiny ornaments, getting ready for Christmas Day. The sitting geese began quacking, and must not have seen me because they started following my sister past Auntie Qose and her sister Auntie Nancy's house. She was terrified and began walking faster, with the geese tailing her in a single line. I counted nine, and my sister was not asking for help but walking with her head stiff and fixed to her destination ahead. I trailed behind the last goose as Ncuncu led all of us, walking fast and crying softly to our house, a distance of less than a quarter mile. She stepped inside the verandah, only to have the geese pour in. She opened the front door, slipped in, and slammed it shut, panting heavily from fast-walking and panic. From outside, I could hear her bawling as she burst into a scream. There was no gate or fence, and the geese were accustomed to just sitting down, filling up our small but cool verandah, hiding in the shade to escape the scorching sun. If we gave them drinking water, they wouldn't stop goose-talking and pooping. We would have to clean it up unless they were chased out. When they came around, Mama would bring out a bowl of bread crumbs or cornmeal, sprinkle it on the dry grass, and dash back in. Through the verandah windows Ncuncu and I watched as the geese, yellow feet and knees unbended, walked back to their house after their feast. She had stopped crying, and we each enjoyed red and white striped Christmas candy canes flavored with peppermint that Mom had brought from the city.

Christmas was a few days away, and soon, we would watch the sun dance, ringing in joy and celebration throughout the village. Our older siblings and cousins were rehearsing their parts for the village nativity drama on the story of the birth of Jesus. Mary and Joseph, the three kings, the glamorous gifts, new clothes to wear, and plenty of food to eat. The community was vibrant with track and field sports, soccer, and a whole community choir. Posh played Uncle Madoda's piano, and we all took turns learning how to masterfully lift and play the heavy accordion. Once in a while, a huge truck came along with a massive movie screen from which the entire village community, sprawled out on the grass on a warm summer Saturday evening, watched American cowboy films sponsored by Boss Taylor, the local white colonial shopkeeper. We ate bean soup, steamed corn bread, fresh peaches, boiled or roasted corn on the cob, guavas, figs, cactus fruit, wild berries, and not much meat, except on rare Sundays.

Our father was a schoolteacher and one of the most educated men in the village. Together with the chief and other men, he held great power and influence and often filled in as a substitute preacher at our local church. He was never home, and on the rare occasions that he returned, my mother never stopped crying. There were no other men to protect my mother and her growing daughters in our household. Since our childhood, we had been familiar with disharmony and lovelessness, accompanied by an unbearable assumption that the separate family units my father established for himself, were happy and supportive of one another.

A formative childhood memory I have carried with me is when we first ran away from our village home with our mother in the middle of the night. Ncuncu was seven years old, and I must have been four. It was dark outside, with a tiny streak of light far away on the horizon that suggested the break of dawn. We ran ahead of our mother, who was balancing a suitcase on her head and a bag in each of her hands. We hurried along a footpath over the mountain and the flatland that separated my home from the bus stop, a distance of approximately three miles.

As the bus approached from a hill a mile away, my mother quickly put me on her back, secured me with a kanga wrapped around her waist, and slung one of the bags over Ncuncu's shoulder to carry into the bus. She could not afford bus fare for all of us, and we were running away in the cover of the dark from our father, who was not even at home. We had to avoid the village gaze, the cold, questioning stares of those watching the forbidden escape. The same village community had witnessed our big mansion stripped empty when a store truck came to load up our repossessed furniture. We learned that our father was arriving on that day from his girlfriend's village, and our mother's flight was an act of self-liberation and emancipation from the shackles of an unhappy marriage. She had often had a spear thrown at her from across the room or a gun pointed at her during heated arguments with her cheating husband. The archangel of protection must have grabbed that weapon every time, or she could have left us long ago. She lived a life of unabated threats of violence, and running away was an act of emancipation, her way of "talking back" at the structures of cultural oppression, daring to defy her marriage and rewrite her life script, and at the same time give us tools for living life. At that moment, right there in the break of dawn, Ncuncu and I were being socialized into bold, non-submissive women.

We went back and forth between Johannesburg and the

village until we were teenagers. Our childhoods were completely disrupted by our father's extra-marital activities. Each time we returned to Johannesburg, we would have to move house, running and hiding from him within Soweto's townships, and he always came after us even as his side families were expanding. We shared a room with our mother, and Ncuncu and I shared a twin bed. Evenings and early mornings, we prayed together. We were Xhosa; our mother did not have a husband by her side to qualify her for a "match-box" house in the urban areas, and the government was relocating Africans to Bantustans to implement its apartheid homeland policy. Displacement and marginality were beginning to set in, shaping our lives and personalities in irreversible ways.

When Posh, Ncuncu, and I came of age, we all attended the same high school – Healdtown High, a co-ed boarding school in Fort Beaufort. A good number of unshakable stalwarts like Dr. Nelson Mandela and Mr. Robert Sobukwe were illustrious students who shared the educational legacy of my alma mater. Ncuncu did well academically, and Posh shares a memory about a story Ncuncu told on one of their long-distance road trips to the village. It was a double period in her isiXhosa class. Anyone who went to Healdtown knows how grueling and boring a double-period class was. Self-loving teachers didn't want to teach it but had to comply with policy. In this instance, as the story goes, the Xhosa teacher would walk in, sit down at his desk, put his feet up, and say, "Today, we are going to have a l-o-o-ng stretch of Xhosa grammar, ad infinitum, ad nauseam!" It didn't help that the teacher announced it that way. Students were frustrated. This just meant they would have to stomach two whole hours of Xhosa stories like Ingqumbo Yeminyanya, grammar, punctuation, and verb-noun order, and the kids would rather be elsewhere.

"Eish! Yo-o-o," someone said.

"Lord God, what hell of a punishment is this?" Ncuncu would murmur.

At Healdtown, Ncuncu's 'manual' was to deliver mail to individual students seated at long, wooden dinner tables. I served as a bell ringer, waking up in time for the first bell at 5:00 AM, an unpaid job that felt a lot like child labor in its harshness. Often, she clashed with the authorities due to tardiness and the heavy-handed, oppressive overseer role of the Matron. "Ntu, Ntu, Ntu," the Matron would let out a wail from up on the dining hall stage, reading the details of my sister's punishment. "T-e-e-l-a-a!" the fifty-strong dining hall full of girls would complete the sentence in a unanimous call-response routine that put my sister in the spotlight. The Matron would often smack her with a hard slap across the face in front of everyone, a type of corporal punishment that has since been banned throughout South Africa's educational institutions. It was disheartening, but most of the students fully backed and helped her recover from the shock of a disciplinary infraction.

Ncuncu played a mean game of tenniquoit, a circular, frisbee-like rubber ring thrown over a net, and had many friends who adored her and cheered her on. I remember that my sister jumped high up in the air and let out a victory cry before she "placed" the tenniquoit in the opponent's court. "Whoaa-AH!" No one could catch her 'place,' and loud spectator cheers could be heard throughout the court as the opponent composed herself for another attempt at beating her.

It was at this boarding school that my sister taught me how to tie a tie and take pride in my school blazer's badge, Alis velut aquilarum surgent [Latin for: They will soar as if with the wings of eagles]. She taught me how to properly wear my neatly ironed yellow and burgundy school tunic, throw a leg, and make the tunic swoosh in front of the boys' marching brass band whenever you turned the "co-r-r-r-n-e-er!" If it swooshed right, it talked directly to the boy you crushed on. If the one you rejected noticed the swoosh, he could eat his heart out and die or survive; it was his choice. Girls marched to the sound and precision of drumbeat performance along the main street, all the way from eMzana, to join the boys at the Assembly Square before Sunday service. This was a delightful once-a-week occasion that would have anyone released from the sick bay against medical advice just to attend the main service. At the end of my first year, Ncuncu transferred to another school. Before leaving, she worried that I would not survive Healdtown's heavy peer pressure and discover all about dating under the moonlit willow trees of "Avenue." The short strip between Mzana and Mzimkulu was a romantic paradise. She was comforted by the fact that I was thin, scrawny, and flat-chested, and no sensible boy cared to look. For the most part, boys were older and only saw me as a baby. Just recently, Posh and I were chatting about one popular constitutional judge who was my classmate. This man would disappear to smoke a blunt with his friends during 'short-break.' The next class would be filled with extraordinary brilliance as he earned the history teacher's praise for his philosophical arguments. He seemed humble and reserved, and, along with the louder boys, he sat against the wall in the back row of the class. That spot seemed like a throne for future kings. There, they percolated political activism or teased girls with vulgar, except that the 'now judge' constantly reprimanded them for using corrosive language in front of a child, me. "Khanimeni madoda, kukho umntana apha maan." There's a child among us, he would say, looking at me with apologetic eyes. That was the extent of my relationship with the opposite sex. Still, I would never miss a moment to stand along Avenue when a bus full of handsome-looking young men rolled in from Freemantle High for a soccer or rugby match, and all the girls were all over the street screaming, ululating, and hollering, "Freeze, amadod'ethu!" Boarding school was fun.

Our mother, too, was afraid I might be sick because I was sixteen and had not yet been to the moon – not seen my period. So, she began mailing care packages containing Nestle's Klim powdered milk and cans of beans to feed me every kind of protein that could stimulate this process to begin already. Shortly after Ncuncu transferred, I was plumpy, and Mama was comforted. Healdtown was not only a famous school but an institution for socialization into adulthood, a place to learn gendered roles and outgrow the comforts of sleep-ins and apprehensions that come with teenage angst.

Ncuncu enrolled at St. John's College, a boys' school near

Umtata, where she was one of the first and only two girls to integrate into a single-sex school, beginning the process of transforming it into an institution that recognized gender diversity. In the late seventies, she entered the teaching profession in Soweto. She dressed in very expensive clothes and often let me inherit some. She did not like going through the closet to find a dress missing, and she would be upset that I had used it without her permission and did not return it to its wooden hanger.

Ms. PK, her friend, tells the story of massive teachers' walkouts and resignations early in their careers. During the 1976 Soweto Uprising, teachers in Soweto played a crucial role in supporting student protests. Many ignored the government's directive to use Afrikaans as a medium of instruction for mathematics and social science classes. When these teachers refused to comply, they were fired, which further escalated tensions. As the situation intensified, teachers began to resign in protest. With the exodus, teachers wanted to force the apartheid regime to listen to their demands. In response, the government took drastic steps, shut down schools, and expelled striking students and protesting teachers. Students also refused to write papers in Afrikaans and were subsequently expelled from schools. One school after another saw students and teachers going on strike, demanding their right to reject Afrikaans and to teach and be taught in their languages. The teachers' protests and resignations were an integral part of the broader movement against racial injustice and the imposition of Afrikaans. Some teachers faced persecution and imprisonment for their involvement in the protests. The teachers' actions demonstrated their solidarity with the students, and their actions contributed to the crisis of legitimacy faced by the apartheid government and ultimately played a role in its downfall in 1994.

Four months without a salary was exceptionally tough for Ncuncu and Ms. PK, her new friend. They met at Moletsane Secondary School and began searching for employment in other schools. They forged a relationship of support that extended to attending each other's family events. They learned each other's languages of isiXhosa and Setswana, and enrolled for their junior degrees together, with Ncuncu attending Vista University and Ms. PK opting to study with the University of South Africa.

In 1982, Ncuncu and I were fully grown young women when our grandmother, our father's mother, died. We were generally curious to understand the marital schisms, splits, and divisions that persisted and caused strained relationships in our large family. Our mother was already in her sixties and supported by a walking stick, but continued teaching. There were few memories of a happy childhood, and we did not have the blessing of a doting, caring father. Our relationship with him was loveless and based mostly on fear and a demand for deference and respect. As our family grew bigger, new hostilities germinated that dated back to a period when the family patriarch habitually yanked us out of school whenever a new baby came along, turning us into nannies for his extramarital children while we were young kids ourselves.

On the day of our grandmother's burial, my father's three nuclear families were all gathered together for an event that became a significant milestone in the process through which Ncuncu and I would grow into womanhood. Because the most significant man in our family played such a detrimental role, we relied on the support system of women outside the paternal family, drawing strength and courage to understand the workings of an unchallenged patriarchal system of dominance. Briefly, under customary law, in collaboration with distorted apartheid legal structures, African women were treated as minors, even as married women. Among other things, African women could not hold a bank account without the signature of a male guardian and, indeed, had no right to seek a divorce. It was the prerogative of the husband to divorce his wife if he so wished. Until the day she died in 1993, our mother was legally married to our father, even though he had physically and emotionally left the family when we were toddlers. Our father knew that it would be to his economic advantage not to grant the divorce my mother desired. In young adulthood, all his daughters could potentially marry, and he could benefit from the system of lobola. By the time of my brother's death, I had grown so angered by my father's actions, in particular, because my mother had no legal recourse due to her status as a "minor" under the law. Although heroic, it pained us to watch our mother struggle to raise and educate four of us single-handedly. The culture of silence and fear in the family prevented its diverse members from intervening in my mother's treatment and the beatings she was subjected to due to his infidelity. Rather, resentful attitudes and behaviors percolated and were reinforced and reproduced as newer children were born and socialized into old secrets. Growing up in this environment impacted family relationships and led to more tension, anxiety, and stress-related behaviors.

Our late brother had become aware of differential treatment in the mixed family and, in his youth, developed an urgent impulse to protect us. It was on this funeral occasion that we had an opportunity to witness him in that role. My father had summoned me into a separate "hut" where he was set to punish me for an altercation on the food line. I recall that my sister informed my brother and members of my nucleus and I saw him approach the patriarch, armed with a rock like David in the face of Goliath. "Tsiba," my brother commanded me to jump over the lower portion of the two-part wooden door. It was locked, and my brother knew that I was trapped, and I was about to be killed by a ferocious man. There was much excitement at this point, but soon, the older man gave up the quest of killing his daughter as the youthful son approached and vehemently defended a powerless female sibling. My sister comforted me, and my brother took me by the hand and led me to my mother's side. I sat on the bed, with my head on my mother's lap, shocked and sobbing. There was a soft knock, and Mom balanced herself with her walking stick towards the locked door to receive food that my sister Ncuncu had brought. She closed the door of the room and never again mentioned what had happened. The lines had been drawn, and the polarized relations in the three families were reaffirmed.

Ncuncu had grown a close-knit relationship with all her siblings, with an even closer kinship with our only brother. In his youth, my 6'1" brother had a towering presence in our family of five, and we relied on him as a source of comfort and a voice of reason that mediated little disputes among us. He had somehow picked up the nickname "Jan van Riebeeck," after the notorious Dutch colonizer, because of a position he played as a school soccer coach that had him display an imposing stature, invade, take up space, and control the ball, subjugating it like a native under his feet. When he was killed by a white man in Parys, a small town in Free State Province, Ncuncu cried until she had isingqala. She wept with all her being, her soul wounded and her spirit visibly shaken. It was an unusual cry that I had never heard before. There was no way of consoling her. They lived together in Protea North, and both loved cooking large, healthy Sunday dinners, and hosting a few of their friends on weekends. He raised her son, my sister Posh's daughter, and my older son and often took the boys to Orlando Stadium to watch Kaiser Chiefs play against Moroka Swallows or Orlando Pirates. They had many boy stories to tell over a dinner of amadombolo, morogo, and curried lamb. On those days, Ncuncu's four-room house was filled with the smell of fresh food, sweat, and sometimes beer. Ncuncu would always be at the center of those men's discussions, interrupting or moderating them, even though she had not been to the stadium.

Ncuncu had a genuine and inborn love for children that was evident to us at an early age, and it led her away from a career path in nursing, which she began in Port Elizabeth right after high school. She had a quality of empathy and nurturing that could have turned her into Florence Nightingale herself. But she had been born into a family of teachers, so it was not surprising that she remained in that profession for thirty years, transferring this skill into the classroom and, ultimately, into educational leadership.

Ncuncu's career path was not so different from mine. I had begun as a promising nurse but ended up in the teaching profession by default, derailed by South Africa's system of arbitrary political detention. The year was 1984. After my release from a cold, mountain-top prison in Harrismith, KwaZulu-Natal, Zi took me by the hand into her mother's bedroom and pleaded with her to help me leave South Africa.

We were neighbors. I lived with my uncle MacKay, two streets away from the original Mandela family's modest four-roomed house on Vilakazi Street in Orlando West. Through an exiled friend, Dumakude, son of MaNkosi, I had been accepted to Hunter College in New York. But I had no means, no passport, and no hope. The apartheid government had barred me from traveling abroad "until further notice," and my Transkei booklet—essentially a passport for Bantustan citizens—could only get me as far as Swaziland, Botswana, or Lesotho. "But darling, you know we can barely survive. How will I be able to do this?" Auntie Winnie asked, her voice heavy with concern. "Mommy, take a good look at her, please. It's a small amount. Look at the travel agent's invoice," Zi urged.

Sitting at the foot of Auntie Winnie's bed, I overheard their intimate mother-daughter exchange. My heart pounded, my bare toes curled against my open sandals, and numbness set in as tears streamed down my face. Somehow, Zi—whom I had known only as my boyfriend's friend—moved her mother to compassion. Auntie Winnie's heart softened, and she decided to help me.

She walked me to the low-fenced gate past Khruschev, the family's lion dog named after Nikita Khrushchev. The dog sniffed my toes but didn't bark. "Don't pat him. Walk slowly beside me, and you'll be fine," Zi cautioned. "Bye. I'll send a child to Uncle Mackay's," she said as I pulled the gate toward me and watched Khruschev retreat to his doghouse.

A few days later, a child I didn't recognize knocked at our door, handing me an envelope. Inside was a check with my name on it, covering the exact shortfall that had separated me from my dream. That check, a fraction of my one-way ticket to New York, was from Auntie Winnie Nomzamo Mandela. The larger contribution came from a company called Hewlett-Packard. Both women are no longer with us, but their selfless compassion and commitment to justice, freedom, and democracy left an indelible mark on me. They strengthened my resolve to fight for human rights, both within and beyond my country's borders.

When I returned to my uncle's home after several months of detention, I knew I was lucky. Many Black South Africans never made it out of prison alive. Stories of torture, rape, and death abounded— men and women "falling" from windows or "slipping" on soap in showers. It was a time when young Black people were trapped in a web of suspicion, interrogated about their connections to political leaders.

My imprisonment was just such an experience. One fateful day, I was returning home to Soweto after being fired from a pharmaceutical job six hundred miles away. My employer had sent me to market infant formula as a human milk substitute. When I discovered its significant nutritional shortcomings, I shifted my workshops to advocate for breastfeeding instead. The company retaliated, repossessing my car and leaving me stranded, unable to pay rent. Desperate, I hitchhiked on the N3 freeway. My final ride dropped me off in Harrismith, where I stopped at a restaurant, unknowingly entering through a "Whites Only" door. The actual entrance for Black patrons was a tiny, burglar-proofed window at the back. The white cashier immediately called the police. Moments later, four officers entered the restaurant. I heard one say, "Die kaffirvrou met 'n rooi kap" - "The n-word woman with a red hat." To the delight of the white patrons, the police conducted a humiliating public search. A small SWAPO brooch pinned to my hat had triggered their paranoia. Inside my bag, they found banned literature—books about slavery, Jim Crow laws, and the liberation struggles of African Americans. Among them was a book titled Call Me Not a Man by a South African author, also banned.

Under the law, I should have been exonerated; the books were for personal use, not distribution. But justice for Black South Africans was elusive. I was arrested and detained without trial in a maximum-security prison—for reading about racism and liberation. Imprisonment left me seething with anger. Denied the right to a lawyer, I was stripped of my basic human rights. The injustice of my detention compounded the deep rage I carried. Yet outwardly, I remained motionless and pleasant, a mask that concealed the storm within.

Months after my release, my application for a passport to travel to the United States—where I had been accepted to pursue a bachelor's degree at a four-year college—was denied. I was forced to wait another year. The official rationale was rooted in my ethnicity: as a Xhosa, I was deemed ineligible for a South African passport, a privilege reserved for white citizens. The homeland policy, designed to fragment and oppress, had caught up with me.

Under apartheid, ethnicity was a weapon wielded by the government to marginalize, subjugate, and exploit Africans within the political economy. It determined where we could live, whom we could marry, and even the extent of our freedom to move.

Eventually, I was granted a passport and, with it, the chance to break free. My escape was made possible through the support of a multinational corporation that played a vital role in the international divestment movement—a global effort to pressure and isolate South Africa's apartheid regime through economic sanctions. Winnie Nomzamo Mandela, known to the world as the Mother of the Nation, also played a pivotal role in my journey to higher education. As the wife of South Africa's first Black president, her compassion and advocacy became a pathway for my dreams. Years later, armed with a doctorate and a determination to serve my country, I found myself working at the Union Buildings in President Nelson Mandela's administration. I served as a race and gender policy researcher, helping lay the groundwork for the establishment of the Office on the Status of Women in the Presidency.

III

The Diagnosis and Its Impact

The urgency in the ringing analog phone line echoed through the hotel lobby. It was my son calling from downstairs. Ncuncu and I had been anxiously expecting the call. Flinging my cell phone on the bed, I rushed out of the room, bypassed the elevator, and took 'double-up' steps to the first floor. The airport-rented family-size truck awaited me at the entrance, the door wide open. My two sons and granddaughter looked weary from their long road trip from New York City. The scorching day beat down upon us as we gathered in front of the hotel, having traveled from California and The Bronx to this meeting point outside Boston, Massachusetts. Ncuncu had joined a group of educators for a course on school leadership at Harvard University, and we needed to come to greet her and pray together. She had encountered some professional challenges, but her legacy as a school principal flourished. Her students soared and achieved matriculation standards that defied racial stereotypes about the academic performance of Black students in Soweto. Building on the excellence of the school principal before her, she produced top graduation results for her school region, and she was invited to Harvard University in Massachusetts. As an educator, she was accustomed to traveling abroad, sharing instructional best practices, and learning about educational systems in Eastern and Western European settings. For her, the Harvard invitation was important because it coincided with her diagnosis. She was shocked and rattled by the news but put on a brave face and traveled to Boston.

Family is important to us, so my children were obliged. As we locked the vehicle doors, the four of us filled the hot elevator, headed upstairs, and impatiently knocked on the room door.

"Auntie-e-e, open this d-o-o-r-r!"

"Come in, it's open." The door swung open. Ncuncu was on her feet, welcoming the crew. We both broke out into a spontaneous call-response poem, a nursery rhyme of our childhood.

Ncuncu: "Ngubani na lo?"

Me: "Ngu Yeye"

Ncuncu: "Uhamba nabani?"

Me: "NoYise"

Ncuncu: "Umphathele ntoni?"

Me: "Amasi"

Ncuncu: "Ngendeb'enjani?"

Me: "Ebomvu!"

My adult sons didn't catch that one, not even my older Xennial son, a fascinating microgeneration that straddles the line between Gen X and Millennials. It was a kindergarten poem far removed from his generation. Ncuncu walked closer to them, with her signature half smile, half laugh on her face.

"Say hello, Auntie," Bubu instructed Boni-Boni.

"Hello, Auntie," Boni said to Ncuncu, hiding behind her father's head, her arms clasped tightly around his neck.

"Naa-uh, she's not your Auntie, baby. She's your Gogo." I said, pausing to figure out an appropriate English word to convey the relationship accurately. In times like these, the English language can be deficient. Before I could finish contemplating, I heard, "Hello, Auntie Gogo." In her innocence, Boni-Boni had unwittingly invented a new kinship term. At that precious moment, the room was filled with my sister's laughter of pure joy as she began to teketisa the toddler like a typical Xhosa mother.

"Yhuu. Ngubani na lo nongcathalalana?" She asked, this time referencing a skinny Disney character in isiXhosa. "iYhoo, matse matse matse," and she pulled the little girl perched high on her father's shoulders into her arms.

"What's your name?" "How old are you?" Boni-Boni loosened her grip, slid down willingly, settled in, and rested her head on Ncuncu's chest with her thumb in her mouth. She was tickled. They were both searching each other's foreheads and touching faces as they shared a tender exchange. For a moment, Boni-Boni was carefully touching Ncuncu's left hand but didn't say anything. Ncuncu was born with syndactyly, a webbing of her left ring and middle fingers, which never got surgically separated.

"Boni-Boni, and I'm four." She said, with a display of four fingers in between her and Ncuncu's faces.

"Really? That's your great-grandmother's name. Boniswa and you look just like her. Your name means the one with the gift of sight, the visionary, the one who sees what others don't see and can't see." That made Boni-Boni squish her eyes tightly.

Ncuncu didn't show any signs of anxiety or fear but spoke with her usual confidence and self-assurance. "I briefed my roommate, so she's aware that you're coming to stay with me for a week. We'll sleep in my bed, and you can stay and rest when I'm in class."

"That's alright, I'm on summer break and not teaching until the fall, in September."

"Vi, O my goodness, you're so grown." My sister was reading the room, greeting and acknowledging all of us, one by one.

"Yea. It's been a long time, Auntie."

"I'm thirsty, Dad." There was water in the hotel fridge, so I walked over, brought out four bottles and we sat on the couch and on Ncuncu's bed, chatted, and walked down memory lane. Bubu had been raised by his grandmother, our mother Boniswa, so there were many stories to share about our home in Butterworth. The beautiful garden grandma kept and tilled with her own hands, cultivating and harvesting pumpkins, beetroots, carrots, cabbages, spinach, and sunflowers that grew so tall they covered the back windows of our house like yellow curtains. As our mother's first grandchild, Bubu lived with her for a few years in our Butterworth home. He told us how terrified he was of the tiny garden snakes and earthworms in that garden that gave him nightmares in his childhood. My family, together, all exhausted from a long flight from California, a long drive from New York City, and a 22-hour long flight from South Africa, and this small hotel room felt like a sanctuary. We made a brief prayer and chatted some more. It felt like home. My jetlagged sister's roommate must have been overwhelmed because she slept through it. Bubu and Vi left with the toddler late that night, headed to some place in Massachusetts to rest and drive back to New York City the following day.

The next morning started well. An early supper had been scheduled, and tables were bedecked with guests in aprons decorated with gigantic red lobster artwork. Most of the guests were tasting lobster for the first time in their lives, and that included Ncuncu. After a while, they decided not to use the complicated shell-cracking instruments, and a few others had mastered a new skill: pulling the meat out by cracking the shell on the wooden table. Ncuncu and I had almost missed the supper. Earlier on, while getting dressed, she had misplaced her passport and had her handbag contents emptied all over her bed, searching for it. Her roommate was in the shower.

"Asibaxelelanga ke, Dzedze." Ncuncu stated that she did not share the shocking news with the training program organizers. "I would have missed a great opportunity that had been scheduled long before the diagnosis." She was right. There was much at stake, and she had planned to return from this trip, her mind ablaze with new ideas and ready to transform her school.

"Oh. Okay," I replied. "Did you look in your luggage for the passport?" We searched and found the passport lodged and zipped up in the inside pocket of the handbag. After getting dressed, we headed for the elevator and pressed the first-floor button. We landed downstairs and she began searching her pockets and said she forgot to bring the room key. She needed to go back upstairs to get it.

"Where's the lift?"

"It's right behind you, Sisi."

We hopped back in and grabbed one of the electronic cards on the dresser.

"Ngu-dum-ti-ri-ri!" She said it herself. "But I'm getting used to it!"

These missing objects were icebreakers for us to broach the dreaded subject of the diagnosis.

"Akho ngxaki, MaRadebe. "Do not despair, Sisi," I said gently. "We'll ride the storm together. Posh and I are already talking and sharing strategies."

I wasn't sure how reassuring my words sounded, but I didn't want to reinforce nursery rhymes like dumtiriri—the classic kindergarten tale of a large, round egg that perches precariously on a fence, only to fall and shatter. Preschoolers recite such rhymes innocently, unaware of their deeper spiritual undertones. Sitting on the fence of indecision or succumbing to fear often leads to a steep descent into darkness—a loss of purpose and connection as spiritual beings. My sister and I were embarking on a sacred journey—one that called for profound self-knowledge, revelation, and divine guidance to confront the realities of Alzheimer's. We both understood the weight of the commitment and responsibility that lay ahead for all of us. Even in this moment, my sister's metaphorical wit shone through, a reminder of her unique perspective and enduring spirit.

A week later, we hugged, and in that embrace, she told me the group was departing for a tour to some other American city. It was time for me to travel back to The Bronx.

"It is well," I told her. "We'll take it as it comes and read as much as we can to know what to do. God will watch over you every step of the way, and we'll fight it together to the last breath." She thanked me for coming through to be with her, and we promised each other that we would call every Saturday. Wi-Fi is not so good in Kelvin, but I assured her that I would reload my calling card and connect so she wouldn't have to point that slow, old-technology BlackBerry phone in different directions just to catch a signal.

"We will start the first Saturday after you return home when you've recovered from your trip."

"OK, and if I don't remember, remind me. Remember for me, Dzedze," she said, with a broad half smile, half laughter that always exposed four beautiful incisors followed by a missing tooth on each side of her upper jaw. My answer had to be reassuring, or I'd miss the mark. After all, I lived thousands of miles away, in a different country altogether. My heart snapped. I knew that my role in caring for her would have to be different as I pondered what it meant to remember for her.

Ncuncu was diagnosed with Alzheimer's in 2012—the same year she went to Harvard. A week before she traveled, our older sister Posh called to prepare me for the task of informing the rest of our family in the US about the news.

Posh explained how she first noticed the signs. One day, after returning home from Northwest, she found that Ncuncu had been skipping work. When asked why, Ncuncu confessed, "I can't go to work anymore because I forget too easily."

Posh began observing other subtle changes. Small things, like misplacing her keys or handing her debit cards and PINs to random strangers who helped her at the ATM. These behaviors gradually escalated. When the family ultimately decided it was time for her to retire, Ncuncu was serving as a school principal.

Then came the more troubling episodes. She started forgetting her off-ramp on the highway. Each time, she would pull into the nearest petrol station and ask a stranger for help, requesting they drive with her to guide her home.

"We've decided to let her stop working immediately," Posh said in a panicked voice. "This is too dangerous. We cannot let her risk her life like that." I agreed, and soon, she could not drive to Pick N Pay, the local corner store to get bread and milk; she got lost coming back home.

"Begging and convincing her to retire was the hardest thing to do, but she listened to the cautionary tone of the request," Posh said.

As promised, two weekends later, I had my calling card reloaded and sat in front of my local Starbucks so I could catch Wi-Fi and stay connected for the duration of the call.

"Hello Dzedze," her voice told me she was smiling. But the next question surprised me. "Uphi? Are you at the gate? Wait, I'm coming to open the gate for you."

"No, silly. But I will be at the gate soon. I will let you know when I get there. How are you? Are you still jetlagged?"

"Ooh. Ag, nxa. I forgot I left you in Boston." We chatted for a while, and I wanted to say good night so she could get some rest, but I changed the subject and informed her that I would be moving from New York City to California in 2013. We lamented the three-hour time difference. New York had seemed closer to Johannesburg on the clock. Now, the Pacific Time Zone would separate us by another three hours. She had the most difficult phone to operate, a Blackberry, and said she would set up an alert.

"Hayi Dzedze, let's not despair. We can call each other every Saturday around this time," my sister suggested. "I'll know it's you when the phone rings at 20H00. When I can't remember, you will remind me. Haha. No, you will remember for me, mntakamama."

That November, I traveled and visited my family and began what would be an annual pilgrimage to be with them. I booked an airplane ticket, packed my bags, and headed home. It was October 2012, in the middle of the fall semester, when a storm called Hurricane Sandy became ferocious, its effects far-reaching throughout New York, New Jersey, and Connecticut. Classes had to be canceled and converted into asynchronous online modality. I extended deadlines for submission of postgraduate students' final papers and took some on the airplane home to mark and post grades online via Canvas. Our older sister Posh lived and worked in Northwest Province, so I stayed with Ncuncu for a while. That weekend, immediately after my arrival, Ncuncu and I went to the bank in Sandton. We must have sat for an hour, reading long legal documents, across from the mortgage broker, a very kind man. My sister had asked that I accompany her to pay off her house. She said she didn't want complications with monthly payments when her condition worsened. She was preparing ahead of the disease, outsmarting it by a week, a mile, a year, a brainwave, whatever the measure of decline would be, it wasn't going to catch her in deep sleep.

Upon completing her bank formalities, we ventured to Woolies for some shopping. That day, we faced a heart-wrenching ordeal that would later be identified as an early sign of Alzheimer's. The whereabouts of Ncuncu's BMW eluded us in the sprawling parking lot. Hours ticked by as we sought assistance, reaching out to her son in hopes of jogging his memory for the license plate number, but to no avail. Friends were phoned in a bid to pinpoint the model, yet all I could recall was its distinctive silver-grey hue. The parking slip offered no guidance, lacking a bay number or a hint of location, and amidst the sea of vehicles, each seemed a mirror image of a BMW X series. Ncuncu's recollection of her plate and insurance details had faded, leaving us without a lifeline for roadside aid. After a weary trek across numerous bays, mall security extended a helping hand, contacting the BMW dealership on our behalf. Relief arrived in the form of a patrol car, its tracking system reuniting us with the elusive vehicle.

Up until that moment, the quest to locate her car had stretched on, a source of mounting tension for my sister. Her attachment to the vehicle was palpable; it was a recent acquisition, a treasure she was loath to entrust to another's care. The memory of a simpler time lingers - a pause in our journey by the roadside, the aroma of roasted corn on the cob beckoning. Ncuncu signaled our intent to merge onto the bustling main artery of Potchefstroom Road. Yet, the relentless tide of vehicles daunted her. In a rare surrender, she stepped from the car, assuming the role of conductor to the symphony of motion, her arm outstretched, ushering the stream of cars with a firm "Gqitha-a-a-ni! Pass!" She sought an opening in the endless flow, a moment when she could seamlessly weave into the tapestry of traffic. Meanwhile, my offers to navigate the chaos from behind the wheel were met with quiet resignation: "Yhuu hai, imot'wam. Not my car, I'll drive!" My attempts were, but whispers lost in the roar of engines.

These episodes served as a stark reminder of the pressing need for Posh, who had journeyed back to the Northwest to gather her remaining possessions, arrange vital live-in support, and relieve Ncuncu of her driving duties. That summer, we discussed the diagnosis as a family and confirmed among ourselves that traces of a genetic component had been found decades earlier, when our maternal aunt, in the throes of dementia, wandered away from the familiar confines of her home compound, never to return. In the hushed whispers of family lore, her absence lingered as a silent wound, a testament to the unimaginable depths of loss and disconnection brought on by memory disorder. For years, our aunt's whereabouts remained a mystery, her absence a palpable presence that haunted the fringes of our collective consciousness. At family reunions, it was a silent but persistent question, discernible only in the pain-filled eyes of her daughter and adult grandchildren. How could an adult woman disappear for decades without a trace? Where could she have wandered to? No one understood, and none of our family members had an answer to a mystery that lasted upward of two decades.

After twenty years had passed, a glimmer of truth surfaced, illuminating the obscure corners of our history. An assignment was announced for close kin to travel to a village far away to exhume her body and bring it home to her people for proper burial. She had wandered into a family unknown to us that had sheltered her in her twilight years, unaware of her lineage, her history, her very essence. In death, our aunt had found solace in the embrace of strangers, her final resting place an unmarked grave, a silent testament to the unspoken grief that bound us together.

For Ncuncu and our family, the revelation of our aunt's journey with dementia reverberated with profound significance, a mirror reflecting the fragile threads that connect us across time and space. In her diagnosis, Ncuncu saw echoes of our aunt's silent struggle, and it was a haunting reminder of the genetic legacy that binds us to the shadows of the past.

"This means I inherited the gene. Auntie Dani's disease is now my disease." When Ncuncu lamented this way one day, I was left broken. Her words cut deep as they were tinged with sadness and resignation and spoke volumes of the burden we carry—a burden of unspoken grief, of relationships lost and forgotten, and wounds that refuse to heal. Soon enough, the doctors explained the link to family history and stated that having a parent or grandparent with early-onset Alzheimer's increases the risk, but it doesn't guarantee that you will develop the disease. However, it was a maternal aunt that we knew to have some form of dementia, and none of our parents did, so it was extremely confusing to understand the doctor's explanation.

"We will need to take care of her as a team. Lord, Jesus, what will I do?" I was talking to myself, questioning God over and over, wondering about the enormity of caregiving and the fact that my older sisters both lived as single women at the peak of their careers. My academic career was new. I had just begun teaching three classes at the City University of New York, and a graduate course at Columbia University. Only a few years back I had had a budding academic leadership career cut short by a massive merger of three universities in South Africa that sent me packing back to the US to rejoin my young family that I had left behind when I graduated.

"Ncuncu has a comfortable home, and we will provide care for her in her own home." Posh was resolute, and I agreed without hesitation. I had seen too many YouTube videos of institutionalized elderly abuse and read plenty of anecdotes of patients' stories in nursing facilities that confirmed the phenomenon. As a family, we pondered societal perceptions about dementia, and we wanted to shelter in and protect our sister from physical, emotional, and psychic harm. With that settled, arrangements and the rhythm for caregiving responsibilities soon began to unfold.

The diagnosis of Alzheimer's at any age can be distressing and particularly traumatic due to its impact on work, finances, and family. As her short-term memory took a hit, Ncuncu relied on help from others for shopping and was restricted from driving.

She gradually began to be unable to determine bank balance losses, struggled to remember names and ATM PINs, and encountered financial abuse from individuals she had become close with. We got to learn and understand that early onset Alzheimer's presents challenges such as memory loss, especially difficulty remembering recent events and names of people and objects. Other symptoms may include poor judgment, mood changes, and challenges with daily tasks.

"I'm going to begin stem cell treatment. My friend has called the company that will put me on the program and monitor the process." Ncuncu mentioned that on one of our weekend calls.

Determined that the line of communication would never break, we continued to share online crossword puzzles and a few other memory games for people with dementia, making sure we kept routine activities that would occupy her mind. My sister was an English teacher, but when Posh emailed me an illegible letter Ncuncu had written, I was devastated. The word order and sentences were garbled, and there were changes in her writing that showed a lack of syntax and semantic order. Rather than proceeding from the left to the right margin, sentences were written from the top of the page with a downward slant that resembled a cliffhanger. Some letters and words were repeated, and it was clear that language and writing were impacted even at this early stage of the disease.

Various relatives sought to decode the origins of Ncuncu's condition. Her endearing nature had won her widespread affection, prompting a multitude of suggestions for overcoming her condition. Curiously, her diagnosis became entwined with notions of her entering a spiritual vocation as a traditional healer. In response to these speculations, my sister understood our African cultural context but was astute in navigating her intricate web of cultural freedoms. She firmly dismissed this interpretation of the cause of Alzheimer's. Asserting her autonomy, she repudiated the supposed connection that tied her to a realm she neither acknowledged nor endorsed. She would not be defined as a person in need of ukuthwasa and initiated into igqira. She was beginning to deal with the situation more practically. When she was made to follow a long line of extended family members and relatives marching to amagubu, the drumbeat of amagqira, headed to Tsomo River to consult with ancestors about her illness, she wondered where in the mix of our father's family units the cultural ritual of visiting umlambo (a river) originated. Ncuncu knew that our parents would not have opted for such an unfamiliar and unusual intervention. They passed on when she was in her 40s and 50s, respectively, and never once practiced any of it when they were alive. A 'polygamous' family blending introduces multiple cultural traditions and ritual versions that can cause challenges like disagreements and misunderstandings among family members. Harmonizing the diversity of cultural practices, values and religious beliefs can make some feel their identity compromised. It can complicate relationships and create new tensions.

The impact of the diagnosis was also detectable socially. My sister had always been a talkative person, a straight shooter, and the life of every gathering. I still remember her dancing in a circle with a bunch of about eight other women. She had just recently been diagnosed, and I was on another visit home from my teaching job in New York. The occasion was to celebrate our older sister Posh's friend Nandi, an educator who had returned from exile in Ottawa, Canada. Every time my sister circled by me, she'd slap me on the shoulder or command me, using the lyrics of the song the group was performing. "Dumzela, maan!" she said. As the melody looped for the tenth, perhaps the twelfth time, I found myself succumbing to the rhythm of mirth, sprawled out on the floor as laughter seized me. The air was punctuated by the shrill of a whistle, the chime of cowbells tied to dancers' ankles, and the sight of Nandi's daughter, her spear carving arcs in the air. My laughter was self-directed, a gentle chiding at my lack of natural talent, and disjointed attempts to synchronize and fall in step with the group. They had gracefully transitioned to their knees, bodies swaying in the traditional Xhosa tyityimba dance. This dance, a celebration of womanhood, seemed to mock my untrained inability to dance with smooth and fluid grace, my lack of curves rendering me a spectator in this dance of femininity.

The song, "Xa ungenemzin'am, dumzela" was a thrill that reverberated across the suburb, and Ncuncu sang the loudest. She was leading the group of African women, clapping hands, stomping feet, and telling stories through songs that were unintelligible to residents in a white Pretoria suburb. The same was true when she broke out into song when her name was announced on the loudspeaker for her to step up to the front at our niece Kiki's wedding. Stomping feet, clapping hands to provide rhythm, and clasping the speech she was on her way to the podium to deliver, she rumbled from the back of the crowd:

Ndiya'k shiya. Ndiyak' shiya.
Nobunganxib'ilokhwe enegqabi, ndim' uMadam
Nobunganxib'ilokhwe enegqabi, ndim' uMadam
Qal'apha kum, uze ndodeni
Qal'apha kum, uze ndodeni

Short and full of impact, the song is sung primarily by women. It strikes a blow at imaginary and past lovers of the groom. "You have come here in your most colorful, flowery dress seeking my husband's attention. See your life now. I'm the one getting married!" What? All the women, high heels off, were dancing barefoot in agreement with the lyrics. Guests scattered out on the willow tree covered, manicured green lawn of the beautiful country club. No celebrity invited to sing at this wedding. We got this. On these occasions it was difficult to remain a spectator. Umxhentso dance is a source of pride for Xhosa people; with every foot stomping, trembling shoulder movements, accompanying African drumbeat and voices in agreement, you gain a fresh perspective of who you are. You might even enter the 'realms,' a random state of trance. In early onset, Ncuncu was reluctant to mingle with large numbers of people. But in groups like these, my sister felt safe and she was loved. In these moments, a diagnosis was a thing only for medical doctors and dementia researchers to ponder

about.

IV

Posh's Home-Based Care

Posh carved out her existence in the platinum province of Northwest, a landscape defined by mountains and scattered bushveld shrubs. Her fortnights were marked by journeying to Gauteng—a pilgrimage of sorts. The mantle of primary caregiver descended upon her, not as a burden, but as a sacred duty, a ministry to which she was unwittingly anointed. Phozisa—our elder sister, whose name was whispered into existence by our parents, a young couple grappling with the profound loss of Ndiphiwe, their firstborn son. Phozisa, meaning "she who mends the family's broken hearts," was a prophetic instruction, a name that would come to signify her life's work: to bind the fragmented pieces of our family's spirit, mend the fissures with the adhesive of her unwavering spirit, and sculpt from the remnants a mosaic of renewed hope. Unbeknownst to us, her name was a harbinger of the selfless odyssey she would embark upon. Posh's narrative is one of quiet supplication—asking God to grant another year by divine grace, a year of continued vigor and purpose, to fortify her nest egg for the upcoming period of retirement. Her energy remained undiminished, and she wanted to continue to work, yet she knew this chapter was her ultimate calling—her telos.

Years before Ncuncu's diagnosis, when we were still college students, she became a central figure in our lives and rounded us up to purchase a property in Butterworth, comfortable enough for our mom to find peace and rest when she retired at sixty-three years of age. Before then, when mom's frame was already supported with the aid of a walking stick, Posh had moved her in with her, caring for her and providing comfort and restoration to make up for all the time she had lost, all the years that our mother's life had been eaten by the cankerworm, the locust and the caterpillar referenced in the Book of Joel. There were airplane rides from Gauteng to East London and visits to the beach, enjoying seaside arts and crafts, and our mother had discovered a new, lighter life in retirement. She was especially proud to experience in her lifetime the joy of watching Dr. Nelson Mandela released from prison to become the first Black president of our country. Yes, it was the same mother who had cautioned us as young children to "Hush, don't let them hear his name come out of your mouth!" It was true. You could be arrested and imprisoned just for mentioning the name "Mandela!" in a country that relentlessly micro-managed private spaces and made information inaccessible to the Black population, in an attempt to maintain the apartheid government's narrative that diminished this man's stature into a midget-like figure.

After Mom passed on in 1993, Posh became our surrogate mother. She traveled to Hunter College in New York City to attend my graduation at Madison Square Garden. Posh was the one who invited our father to her Sunnyside flat in the early 2000s and arranged for him to rotate to all our homes and spend time bonding with us, so reconciliation and forgiveness could happen before Archangel Gabriel visited. She refused to let us live our adult lives in anger and bitterness, so she initiated and coordinated these visits with intentionality. It had taken decades of alienation, but Posh was determined to sew the pieces of our brokenness together, like a needle and thread, and she expressed great concern for our children growing up with repetitive patterns of family disharmony and unresolved anger.

Posh was a product of the University of Pretoria, the University of South Africa, and Ongoye University in KZN. Armed with a Master's degree in public administration, an Honor's degree in economics and business economics, and a Bachelor of Commerce degree, respectively, she completed her work assignment in the

Northwest Province in 2013 and moved into a position with senior responsibility at the National Department of Health in 2014. Closer to home in Pretoria, she could now take a leap of faith and embark on transferring her skills into full-time home-based caregiving for our sibling. It was a frightening move at first, but the decision came naturally, and it was unanimously accepted throughout the family. There were new things to learn, and she leaned on our collective belief that the key to helping our sister cope better with imminent Alzheimer's symptoms was for the team to learn new ways to respond to new behaviors that would come along with this form of dementia.

In 2014, I had begun to believe that Ncuncu's Alzheimer's was possibly delayed or in remission. It was not a foolish thought because she had considered stem cell therapy. It was triggered by one of our long-distance telephone conversations, checking in. In that call, Ncuncu was more interested in finding out about my children, and she sounded well on the telephone. She said she missed Boni-Boni. I reminded her that the four-year-old she had met two years earlier was now six, and she had tricked me out of my senses.

"Oh! How, what did she do?"

"Oi, I can't even be mad. It was last night, Friday evening. I'm falling asleep on the couch, and I can sense that she's standing somewhere around me. She's waving her hand in front of my semi-shut eyes to make sure I'm not fake sleeping. Then she approaches my left thumb, lifts it, and presses it against the fingerprint touchpad of my phone. "Ting!" the phone alerts me, and before I'm able to waddle out of my sunken couch, I hear the bedroom door shut, and she's settled back in the bed."

"Yhoo nank'u tsotsi!" Ncuncu exclaimed.

"So, did her dad say anything or do something?" My sister was curious more about her nephew's role in this. The one she helped raise. Was he a good parent?

"Ha! I didn't tell him. It's the privilege of being a grandmother to step up and solve that issue and not have to tell everything," I said.

"She was too sweet. In the morning, she came and sat next to me and confessed, "I didn't want to wake you up, Nana." So, that settled the matter, but we did talk about always needing to ask an adult for permission." Ncuncu understood.

By 2015, three years after the diagnosis, my sister was unable to get dressed on her own.

"Akasakwazi unxiba ipantyhose ngoku," Posh voiced a grim concern about the prognosis when she noticed subtle and sometimes overt changes that were taking place.

"Wow, hai shame, kuya kubanzima, but she's so healthy emzimbeni." She explained that they were both getting dressed for an occasion when Ncuncu had attempted to put on her pantyhose and did so successfully on one leg. When she reminded her to put on pantyhose on the other leg as well, she opened a fresh pack of stockings and put on new pantyhose on the other leg, as instructed. The mix-up meant that she ended up dragging an extra unused pantyhose with each leg.

Ncuncu's difficulty with tasks like dressing herself suggested that she was already in Mild Alzheimer's stage, where memory loss and cognitive decline became more pronounced. Being unable to dress properly was a symptom of apraxia, difficulty, or inability to perform purposeful movements, even though the person has the physical ability to do so. In this case, it affected her ability to dress correctly, and Posh suspected that there could be other outward physical manifestations of Alzheimer's dementia, so she alerted her team to take note. She began to consult with healthcare professionals for personalized care for our sister in the home. To ensure the efficient and proper establishment of a system of care, we had to understand Alzheimer's as a complex condition and study its progression and impact on the brain for ourselves so we would be able to make informed and appropriate support and interventions.

Alzheimer's disease tends to develop slowly and gradually worsen over several years. The five stages associated with Alzheimer's disease begin with the Preclinical Stage, which occurs before noticeable symptoms are evident. In the next stage, Mild Cognitive Impairment (MCI), some individuals experience mild memory problems that are noticeable but not severe enough to interfere significantly with daily life. Literature notes that everyone with MCI progresses to Alzheimer's disease. In the third stage, Mild Alzheimer's Disease, memory loss and cognitive decline become more pronounced. Individuals may have difficulty with tasks like dressing themselves, cooking, and driving. In the fourth stage, Moderate Alzheimer's Disease, symptoms worsen, affecting language, reasoning, and social behavior. Individuals may become more confused, suspicious, fearful, and frustrated due to cognitive losses and increased dependence on others. Swearing and name-calling may result from this frustration. In the last, advanced stage, Severe Alzheimer's Disease, individuals require full assistance with daily activities. Movement, personality, and communication are significantly impaired.

Our family's decision to care for Ncuncu at home was also motivated by a need to avoid potential physical abuse in institutionalized facilities. Physical abuse may be the result of structural discrimination in institutionalized settings. In many African communities, including South Africa, it may largely also result from public perception, shrouded in misconception and misunderstanding about dementia in general. With the fastest-growing population of elderly individuals in the world, Africa finds itself confronting dementia as a silent epidemic. In a culture where aging and wisdom are revered, dementia symptoms may often be attributed to old age rather than a medical condition requiring attention and support. Moreover, as experts and researchers in the field declare, there are deeply ingrained beliefs in witchcraft and spiritual causation that further complicate the discourse surrounding dementia in African society. In South Africa, the perception of dementia as a manifestation of witchcraft takes precedence, casting a shadow of fear and suspicion upon those afflicted with the disease and their families. Lack of awareness and education surrounding the condition perpetuates a cycle of neglect and ignorance. As in many patriarchal societies, older women bear the brunt of this stigma, as they become labeled as witches and are subjected to ostracism, physical violence, and even death at the hands of their communities.

For my family, the impact of these cultural beliefs on Ncuncu's journey with dementia could not be negated. The fear of stigma and discrimination loomed large, prompting us to make the strategic decision to shield her from the dangers of institutionalized caregiving fraught with misunderstanding, mistreatment, and underpaid caregivers. Even within the confines of our big family, the shadow of stigma loomed large. As Ncuncu battled the peak of her illness, some relatives neglected to visit and chose absence over facing the harsh reality of dementia. Their absence and sometimes hurtful remarks became an all-too-familiar echo within our kin.

"Uphi u mama wakho?" one adult asked a child at a family reunion in the village.

"Uphaa kula ndlu inalaa makhulu ongu zincane," the child responded, and there was no reprimand of the child's behavior on the part of the parent. These comments were becoming commonplace in the extended family. Such insensitivity highlighted a gap in educating our youth about empathy. The proverbial chickens had come home to roost; despite shifts in family structure, the legacy of emotional harm persisted. Our collective consciousness had yet to embrace emotional intelligence and its profound impact on interpersonal relationships. The saying "hurt people hurt people" had not yet found its way into our family dialogue. We were present for celebrations and sorrows, bearing gifts at imigidi, birthdays, graduations, weddings, and funerals. Yet, we overlooked the crucial need for a framework to teach our children about the emotional wounds that lead to the dehumanization and marginalization of elders. Nationally, the elderly are often seen as a burden, with old age cast as a bleak tunnel, overshadowing the employment prospects of younger people. Instead of recognizing the elderly as a beacon of empathy, compassion, and wisdom, they are often met with derision and humiliation when their cognitive health declines.

In our sister's case, there was an urgent need to protect her from the scourge of stigma. So, we entered into a pact to keep her at home, no matter the cost. Posh was committed to establishing the home-based caregiving system and immediately assumed the task of power of attorney. I was committed to push-back online, on the phone, and twice-a-year visits to provide full-fledged bedside support. Posh began recruiting, vetting talent, undertaking background checks, hiring and training caregivers, and following the guidelines of the Alzheimer's Association quality care, and the country's compliance laws for employment. She ensured that she would hire caregivers willing to live in. They had to reside in neighborhoods closer to Ncuncu's home to allow for easy shift rotation and to avoid burnout.

Posh invested in costly but required Association for Dementia and Alzheimer's of South Africa (ADASA) training for caregivers, but there were endless challenges. These were mostly associated with the variation and progression of Alzheimer's symptoms and practical difficulties with scheduling or developing caregivers' conceptual understanding of the disease. To address these challenges, she implemented innovative solutions that included creating and routinizing personalized care plans for bathing, meals, medications, doctor's visits, and exercises for Ncuncu. There were also memory-enhancing activities, prayers, and recreational routines like going to the park and playing frisbee. The stability of living with familiar caregivers provided consistent physical and emotional support that was noticeable in the trust Ncuncu had in people who were now living full-time at her residence and, therefore, considered part of her family. The COVID-19 pandemic hit, and Posh was extra careful. When I visited, she ensured that I was quarantined directly from the airport and socially distanced for seven days at a local Bed and Breakfast. When overcrowding became a thorny issue in Ncuncu's home, it was quickly resolved with the intervention of a social worker, thus mitigating her vulnerability to virus transmission.

Ncuncu's needs were regularly assessed, and there was

effective coordination with medical professionals, including a wound specialist. A physiotherapist regularly came in to stretch her left arm which had lost range of motion. Posh ensured a safe and comfortable environment, managing medications and daily routines, and this impacted Ncuncu's well-being and that of the family. Resilience was incorporated into her treatment and care from the beginning with the goal of promoting empathy on the part of caregivers and the patient's emotional well-being. Ncuncu also became a day visitor or spent weekends at the local frail facility in the Midstream retirement community for recreation and trail walks, fostering a sense of belonging and community support. A pastor from Ncuncu's church regularly visited and administered Holy Communion, and Posh would make sure our sister was dressed up in her Manyano uniform and that members of her congregation visited and prayed with her. These activities created purpose and meaning as they revolved around significant life transitions.

Home-based caregiving was not without its challenges, and evidence was provided by the gravity of a distressing situation that came to light involving physical abuse. In a tale of betrayal, the person living with Alzheimer's dementia experienced unseen cruelty within the walls of her residence. In the quiet corners of her home, where love and vulnerability had thrived, darkness took root. Posh, our stalwart caregiver, had meticulously crafted a haven for our sister, a sanctuary where compassion flowed freely. Ncuncu was in the moderate state of the disease, and she could still speak but with a diminished vocabulary of no more than ten repetitive words or phrases. She was also experiencing a phase where she was unaware that she violated social norms through foul language, a common, stage-related symptom of Alzheimer's dementia that the patient exhibits even if they never used swear words before. But within those very walls, a sinister presence lurked, masked by the guise of care. The caregiver, nameless and faceless, had motives far removed from empathy. Their eyes, once filled with the promise of a paycheck, now glinted with greed. They pilfered from Ncuncu's possessions—the delicate silk scarves and rare jewelry and the crumpled bills hidden away in drawers. Clothing went missing, and bedsheets disappeared out of the linen closet. But their transgressions extended beyond mere theft.

One weekend, Posh had hired extra help to assist the live-in caregiver. On a cold afternoon, the young woman was surfing the internet during her break and turned her camera phone to capture an incident that bore witness to the unfolding tragedy. She was shocked but bold, and out of a sense of justice for Ncuncu, she secretly forwarded the video footage to Posh. The video revealed a horror that words alone cannot convey. Our sister, robbed of speech by the relentless march of Alzheimer's, bore the brunt of the caregiver's cruelty and wrath. An unexplained bruise had blossomed on her fragile skin, and in that video, her cries—wordless yet piercing— echoed from the couch on which she sat and where the caregiver gave her lashings all over her feet and legs, throughout the dimly lit rooms of the house. The trusted caregiver was also using verbally abusive language, expressing her displeasure and disgust with caregiving chores like feeding and changing our sister. "You're not a baby. Get up and walk! Futhi undithukile, I don't have to put up with you."

In that moment, Posh's role transcended caregiving; she became a sentinel, a protector. Her heart weighed heavy with the knowledge that trust had been shattered within their sanctuary. She confronted the truth—the stark reality that even within the confines of home, evil could take root.

The video on WhatsApp alerted me at 2:00 AM in the Pacific Standard Time Zone. It defied the time difference because I was awake, and I saw it almost in real time.

"You won't believe it, but I want you to watch and call me back." Posh hadn't forewarned me. She was brief and hung up the phone before I could ask what the video was about. What I saw was beyond disturbing. I wept. My sister was crying like a child, soft but loud all at once. I had gone out of my way to financially offset this caregiver's entrepreneurial son, who was struggling to launch his business as a sketch artist, and felt betrayed that she waited for me to leave for her wickedness to come to light.

Posh's discovery of the abuse inflicted upon our sister was a pivotal moment—one that tested her resolve and compassion. When the hidden camera unveiled the caregiver's cruel slaps, Posh's heart clenched in anguish. But she did not falter. Instead, she transformed her grief into action. Armed with irrefutable evidence, Posh confronted the caregiver on that same day. She called around and soon gathered the support of members of the extended family within reach. Her voice, usually gentle, now carried the weight of justice. She demanded answers, her eyes unwavering. "How could you?" she asked, her words echoing through the brightly lit living room, the palm tree waving its green branches on the window panes. Posh's protective instincts flared. She removed Ncuncu from harm's way, ensuring her safety. Simultaneously, she contacted legal authorities, determined to seek justice for the abuse inflicted upon our sister. Swiftly, Posh terminated the caregiver's employment. The betrayal had severed trust irreparably, and there was no way to tell how long she had been beating our sister. She ensured that the individual faced the consequences of their actions—both legally and morally. But the incident took its emotional toll. Behind closed doors, Posh wept. The weight of responsibility pressed upon her—a caregiver burdened by more than physical care. She grappled with conflicting emotions like anger at the abuser, sorrow for Ncuncu's suffering, and determination to prevent further harm. After securing more help, she increased her hours at the local pool and let her aquatic exercises heal and restore balance to her aching frame.

Posh's resilience shone through. She sought counseling for Ncuncu, herself, and her caregiving team, recognizing that psychological wounds ran deeper than bruises. Together, they began the arduous journey toward healing, rebuilding trust, and creating a safer environment. When I returned later in the year, Posh, Ncuncu, and I took the short dirt road trip to Hoogland Health Hydro for gratitude and tranquility. We then embarked on our routine escape to the Wild Coast for more healing, spa treatments, taking selfies with rainbows, bird watching, meditations, mindful eating, and general wellness programs.

Posh's response to the abuse becomes a testament to the strength of the human spirit—the unwavering commitment to protect those entrusted to our care, even when darkness threatens to engulf us. It is a tale of betrayal and firm determination—a testament to the lengths we go to shield our loved ones from harm. When we returned from our trip, our attention was diverted to a cumulonimbus event, a rare waterspout that mesmerized the small town of Cofimvaba, terrifying villagers into a panic about witchcraft in high places, or the possibility of the world ending that same day, and we were not moved or shaken. Nothing could scare us anymore.

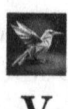

V

Ncuncu's Resilience Transcends Memory

"I'm full!"

That short phrase came out slowly but surely. It didn't sound accidental in its randomness. It was spoken with intentionality and purpose to make me hear very well. I know this because the expression in Ncuncu's eyes matched what she was saying. She wasn't angry because she had that signature smile. Her weary eyes widened as she looked directly into mine and emphasized those two words. I was so stunned that I became drawn to the window behind her, staring outside for a minute and wondering if I had heard right. It was the last time I fed my sister her breakfast. We had returned from our road trip to the Wild Coast, having spent fourteen days of foggy weather, rain, and beautiful rainbows mixed with sun, sand, and good food at Morgan's Bay and Cintsa's Crawford Beach in our home province.

The hardest thing about this trip was feeding our sister. It was raining hard on our final lap home to Pretoria from the Dawn suburb in East London. We stopped at several spots for refreshments, and Posh deliberately avoided our usual freshly baked amagwinya and bypassed that vetkoek shop near Bloemfontein like she didn't see it. Ncuncu would not have been able to enjoy them with us, so there was no point pulling over. She could only tolerate yogurt and a few grapes and slept most of the entire trip. The heavens were thundering, lightning, and beginning to rain hard when we pulled up in front of the door, and every street on Heritage Estate was drenched with tiny rivers of rainwater rushing into drainpipes. I had to hurry ahead and cover every mirror in the house with towels and sheets. Offloading the vehicle was challenging, so we called on gate security for extra help. Just as soon as we locked the front door behind him, load-shedding launched us into darkness, and the struggle began again to make sure Ncuncu ate before bed. We had bright LED lamps for light and soon got ourselves ready for the task.

That following morning, Posh had gone to pick up Dee, Ncuncu's caregiver, from the taxi rank at Grey Owl Shopping Center, and we would prepare her for a doctor's visit. How would I tell the story of Ncuncu's "I'm full" statement without gaslighting myself? Would Posh even believe what I said? Ncuncu had not spoken for a long, long time. She was happy, well-rested, and laughing with us when we took selfies on the fourteenth of December, her birthday, and as usual, she led the conversation and ate a little of her dinner and extra birthday dessert. I made her sit upright on the bed, propped up with plenty of pillows on both sides and her back. I brought in some hot Rooibos tea and her sippy cup of oatmeal, which had been made drinkable. Two to three spoons of tea later, we switched to oatmeal. Ncuncu would not have it. She had not even swallowed the tea; I could see it from her bulging cheeks. I begged and pleaded. The tea trickled out through the corners of her mouth, and I wiped it off. She turned her head to the right, towards the bedroom wall. I brought the spoon close to her mouth again, and she turned her head to the left, towards the dresser with three folding mirrors, still covered in towels from the previous night's lightning bolts. This struck me as strange; something was very wrong. Ncuncu had refused to eat long enough. My next strategy was to sing, "My bonnie lass, she smileth." She did not smile at all. I then decided to call her by her iziduko, the praise names of our Xhosa clan.

"Yitya kaloku, maRadebe, ndlebentle zombini, maShwabada, Aah, Hlubikazi, nceda mntakamama." Ncuncu looked me straight in the eye with the smile I had seen when she was in pain. She took her time to say it. "I'm fu-u-u-ll." Yo! 'Skendabhideka. Her eyes were glazed, and they seemed like they were not blinking. I remembered that when she could still speak, if she was annoyed, she would say, "Khandiyeke maan. Why are you all so busy with me? Mane nindijika jika, nindi duva-duva?" I even missed the time when she would straight up cuss, "Phexe phexe," or sometimes, "Phaxa phaxa ndini. Hamba maan, su-u-ka-a!" She would laugh at me as I walked away to give her space, and I would laugh back, feeling like a happy "gxadada" again.

The way she said those two words had a finality to it. I took it to mean she will never eat again, ever. All I could tell was that something with her swallowing was amiss, like a throat that was too dry to let anything pass into the stomach. Her teeth were clenched, and I would not have had the professional expertise to tell what was wrong, even if she opened her mouth. 'What's blocking her throat from swallowing ordinary tea?' I asked myself. I could not hold my tears. I began to pray, calling on the angels to come feed my sister. I put the cup on the mobile breakfast table, stepped outside the room, and prayed some more, louder, bubbling in tongues, clapping hands and summoning the presence of the Holy Spirit, pacing and moving to and fro. This was more serious than I had thought. I was not panicked, but I needed an immediate answer. I dialed Posh, and her phone rang inside the house, on her bed. Lord, I said to myself, 'She left it behind, and I don't have Dee's number. I'm alone, and this cannot be.' I came right back in, removed all the pillow props, and laid her down on the side. She had had a bath, but her fresh clothes still lay stretched out on the ironing board. When Posh arrived, I had finished getting her dressed in her trek suit, and she was ready to go. We were sitting side by side on the bed, my arm around her, talking to her, telling her how much she meant to me and why we had to believe, together, that everything would be alright. Her face pressed against mine; I could hear her breathing lightly. Her left hand, which used to have a strong grip on it, was trembling as it rested in mine. I was taken aback by the fact that my sister was surprisingly healthy and strong despite Alzheimer's; maybe because of it – how would I know? Not a flu or a cold, and every version of COVID-19 breezed right past her. Her blood pressure, which we checked every day, was better than mine and Posh's. What could it be? As we waited, a long tear rolled down one side of her face. I wiped it off with my hand and said, "Ungalili maRadebe. Don't cry. I'm here. Ungakhali Sisi, uyeva?"

"Ewe, tata!" she replied. I wasn't going to be surprised by that reference. My sister had just made another full sentence, and I allowed myself to be perfectly fine with her responding with a "Yes, Daddy." We sat and waited, reading from Psalm 41, and soon enough, Posh and Dee came in.

"Posh, we need to rush her to the doctor immediately. I think we have an emergency on our hands. Please, let's not even wait to do anything else."

"What happened?" Posh asked. I told her some unusual things happened this morning. When I sat Ncuncu up, she fell on one side like a rock. I propped her up again, and she fell on the other side like a rock. She had become so weak she couldn't sit up without support anymore. Up until then, all through the road trip, she sat up on the bed and supported her frame.

Dee rushed the wheelchair in, and the two escorted Ncuncu to the doctor. I remained behind, in prayer, waiting for the repairman to come in and fix the fridge that had been dysfunctional since we returned from our trip. Essential food items were submerged in a bucketful of ice, melting fast. 'If he can arrive now and get it fixed while the electricity is back from being rationed by the government, we can manage to keep fresh supplies of Ncuncu's favorite yogurt and grapes,' I thought.

My intuition proved correct. The time for yogurt, or any food or drink, had passed for my sister. With a blood sugar level of 3, she was hypoglycemic, and the doctor warned of a potential aspiration risk. Her clenched teeth and refusal of tea and yogurt were her body's defenses against it. That very afternoon, Ncuncu was swiftly taken to the emergency room for immediate surgery. A skilled surgeon was summoned to secure a suitable vein for an IV, to hydrate and strengthen her, and to prepare her for tube feeding.

Reflecting on the journey that began upon our return from the Wild Coast, we now delve into the essence of a beautiful life—a question posed in the opening chapters. Looking back, our singular focus was to provide compassionate care and comfort at our sister's bedside. The initiation of tube feeding, a life-sustaining procedure, marked a pivotal change in our caregiving dynamic as we navigated the twilight of her life. In our dedicated yet narrow approach, we overlooked the breadth of Ncuncu's cognitive abilities, which extended far beyond mere memory retention. This realization dawned on us with great clarity.

As we contemplate the complexities of cognitive function in Alzheimer's beyond the realm of memory, we now consider three critical aspects we came across in the literature in the context of Ncuncu's experience: the nuances of emotional and behavioral shifts, the integrity of sensory and motor pathways, and the preservation of executive function and adaptability. These elements are said to offer a broader perspective on the cognitive landscape affected by Alzheimer's, challenging us to reevaluate our understanding of the disease.

In the realm of sensory and motor integrity, contemporary studies indicate that the neural alterations associated with Alzheimer's extend their influence on sensory and motor functions, surpassing the confines of memory and focus. Ncuncu's capacity for sensory perception and physical response remained remarkably intact. As previously noted, throughout the mild and moderate stages of Alzheimer's, her affinity for music, art, and physical engagement endured despite the encroachment of memory loss. When immersed in Mozart, Beethoven, or Handel's compositions, choral music, and opera, musical experiences she had enjoyed from Healdtown's impeccable chapel choir many years before, her forehead would crease in concentration, and her gaze would brighten. Perched on her bed, she might sway gently or nod to the rhythm, hum softly, or clasp the armrest of her wheelchair firmly as if to physically grasp the notes resonating through her. Her left arm, however, betrayed a growing frailty.

The interlude preceding the peg tube procedure and the events that unfolded served as a period of revelation, profoundly altering our communication with our sister. In the quiet moments that enveloped us as we grappled with the erosion of our known world, Ncuncu imparted an invaluable teaching—one that eclipsed the mere act of remembering. As the disease's hold intensified, she would gaze at us, seeking solace, and murmur, "You will remind me." These words, simple in form, bore immense significance. They beckoned us to bear witness to an unyielding spirit, to the quintessence of life liberated from the shackles of recollection. For a few months, she walked on tiptoe, and she gripped tightly onto her supportive companion, scared that she might fall. It was getting more and more difficult to undertake her daily exercises. We knew that she was in the moderate stage, and we observed great muscle rigidity and witnessed abnormal, jerk-like reflexes and a general decline in physical abilities in those months. Yet, she moved through her environment with an effortless grace, delineating the world's texture with a steady certainty. Sensory and motor faculties we once overlooked as caregivers seemed to emerge as her unspoken confederates. The melody of a cherished tune, for example, would prompt her foot to tap in sync, her eyes to light up in recognition. A gentle touch would coax forth a smile, a testament to a bond that withstood the ravages of cognitive decline. Her eyes sealed shut, her features pulled tight, and her arms no longer raised in exultation, yet her smile, tinged with a poignant depth, assured us that the essence of Handel's Messiah remained indelibly etched within her. In such instances, she illuminated the truth that our being transcends the act of memory.

Emotional and behavioral changes have painted another canvas of complexity. A few anecdotes reveal that our sister's emotional responses have evolved. These demonstrate her emotional resilience, and they include moments of joy, frustration, and connection with loved ones. Anguish and joy dance together, twirling in a delicate balance. When the sun dips below the horizon, our sister gazes out the sliding glass door and notices small birds drinking water from the birdbath, her face a reflection of wonder. And when frustration threatens to overwhelm her, she clasps her hands tightly, seeking solace in touch. At night, speaking in a whisper, she would do the same. Her laughter, unburdened by the past, echoes throughout Posh's home, a flicker of hope.

When the abuse occurred at her own house in Kelvin, she was already in her stage of silence due to linguistic decline. The video shows her attempt to draw attention to the abuser. She screams, and words do not come out of her mouth, but the footage reveals that she is fighting for her life and that she is fully aware that what the caregiver is doing is an abusive infringement of her human right to dignity and safety from harm.

A second illustration of these changes is in order. My sister liked to repeat her name as if she were afraid to forget it. "My name is Smileth," "I am Ncunyiswa Ntutela. Smileth!" she would say. Or, mimicking a classroom roster call, if you called her name, she would reply, "Present!" Repetitive behaviors, such as repeatedly stating one's name or responding to a roll call with "Present!" are common in individuals with Alzheimer's disease. This repetition often stems from a need for comfort, security, and familiarity as the disease progresses and affects the brain's ability to make sense of the world. Memory loss may lead a person to forget recent actions or words, prompting them to repeat themselves, possibly as a way to hold onto their identity. The repetition of her name and response, "Present!" fits like a glove in the area of nuances of emotional and behavioral shifts. This aspect of cognitive function in Alzheimer's disease encompasses changes in behavior and emotional responses that are not solely related to memory. It includes how individuals with Alzheimer's seek to maintain their identity, find comfort in familiarity, and express their needs or emotions through repetitive actions or words. While memory loss is a significant part of Alzheimer's, the disease also affects behavior and emotional regulation. Repeating her name or affirming her presence by saying "Present!" can be seen as a way for Ncuncu to assert her identity and cope with the changes she is experiencing. It is a behavioral adaptation to the cognitive decline, providing her with a sense of control and self-assurance in a world that is becoming increasingly unfamiliar. And then there was executive functioning, that intricate web of decisions and adaptations.

Executive functioning refers to a set of high-level cognitive skills that allow us to plan, organize, carry out, and complete tasks efficiently. It involves self-monitoring, decision-making, and goal-directed behavior. In her article, "How Executive Functioning Is Affected by Dementia," Hereema (2023) writes that in people with Alzheimer's disease, executive functioning is significantly affected, especially as the disease progresses, and that challenging behaviors often associated with Alzheimer's may be related to problems in executive functioning. Hereema says executive functioning impairments may make it seem like the person is behaving selfishly, especially if their memory is still quite intact (ibid). Also of note, while memory impairment often accompanies executive impairment, it's possible for someone to have no memory issues but still struggle with decision-making and executive tasks. Executive function is closely connected to working memory, which plays a role in holding and manipulating information temporarily. Examples of impaired executive functioning in dementia include poor judgment. Individuals may make decisions that seem illogical or risky. The second example is disorganization. Patients exhibit difficulty organizing tasks or managing daily activities. In the third example - socially inappropriate behavior - they demonstrate behaviors that don't align with social norms. Fourthly, they have planning difficulties. They struggle to make plans for events later in the day. Lastly, they have a lack of awareness, failing to note or understand that their behavior affects others.

Ncuncu exhibited all of the examples outlined above. However, we also encountered many moments when she demonstrated resourcefulness or creative problem-solving, suggesting that cognitive resilience extends beyond memory. Ncuncu had difficulty managing daily activities. As we mentioned in another chapter, our sister had a challenge with dressing herself. Early in the diagnosis, certain daily activities like cooking and driving had to be curtailed due to the danger associated with them. As Hereema states, impaired executive functioning can impact multi-step processes like cooking or driving, so precautions are essential in those areas when dealing with dementia. Socially inappropriate behaviors that don't align with social norms were exemplified by excessive cussing, with expletive content framed in the Xhosa language, our mother tongue. Dementia can lead to a loss of inhibition, causing words that would typically be filtered out to be spoken freely. When she encountered physical abuse, the caregiver reported that she had called her names. This put my sister at risk of more abuse for failing to understand how that behavior affected others. This demonstrates that in the area of emotional and behavioral changes, Alzheimer's affects not only memory but also emotions and behavior. The actions of the abusive caregiver reflected a lack of ability to recognize triggers. Mimicking Ncuncu and raising her voice above that of the patient meant that the caregiver was unable to avoid circumstances that provoked swearing. She was a caregiver willfully participating in a socially inappropriate behavior out of the patient's control. Redirecting the caregiver to another task distracted Ncuncu and shifted focus to something a bit more calming.

Poor judgment was the most hazardous in the area of executive functioning because it happened early in the diagnosis. Pulling over at gas stations, for example, and asking random people to help her find her way home was detrimental to her physical safety, as was sharing her ATM PINs with caregivers and drivers, which negatively impacted her financial security. Posh observed that Ncuncu shopped at Woolies by herself early in the diagnosis and once came home with two of the same double-breasted blazers that she liked, only to find a third one hanging in the closet. This all pointed to poor judgment.

Despite memory loss, however, Alzheimer's patients can sometimes surprise us with their ability to adapt and find alternative ways to accomplish daily activities. This was a major observation that we made in the broad category of executive functioning. For example, when she was unable to respond to a question about how she felt, she would lower her head or drop her chin to her chest, prompting you to dig deeper into that nonverbal cue. As already mentioned, she was able to clench her teeth to avoid aspiration when she lost her swallowing reflex. In a very bold, surprise move to avoid being force-fed, she went ahead and stated that she was "full," thus protecting herself from what could have been an outcome of great calamity.

My sister would fold her laundry, straighten up her clothes on the bed, or rearrange photos in Posh's picture album, creating her symphony of shapes and colors. It was not easy to assess how she performed on the crossword puzzles and memory games we shared online as it became difficult for her to manipulate electronic devices. Early on, when she was restricted from cooking but keen to participate in the household activities, Posh and I enjoyed watching her towel dry clean plates, dishes, and utensils, grouping similar things and leaving them on the kitchen counter arranged in order, sometimes in disarray. Now, in her advanced stage of Alzheimer's, before the peg surgery, when hunger tugged at her, she'd find a way—whether it meant pointing to the kitchen or uttering the word "kutya," or "nyum, nyum," miming the act of eating.

As I lay down the pen to close this chapter, I realize that Ncuncu's legacy lies not in the memories we hold for her but in the moments that she gifts us—the ones that defy forgetting. Life, she whispers, is wholesome, even without memory. Assessments or medical labels do not bind her resilience; they flow from an inner wellspring of determination. And so, six months into the surgery, the distinction between her memories and our role as custodians of her essence is clearer. We no longer need to remember for our sister; she reminds us instead to cherish the present, to find beauty in the fragments, and to honor the resilience that transcends mere recollection.

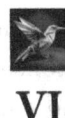

VI

Destigmatizing and Humanizing Alzheimer's Dementia: A Call to Action

We must now look at ways in which Alzheimer's is stigmatized in society, a significant issue that affects both individuals living with dementia and their caregivers. Stigmatization refers to the process by which a mark or attribute—culturally perceived as devalued and discrediting—is recognized in or applied to an individual or group by a more powerful group. This process often leads to negative labeling, exclusion, and discrimination based on perceived differences or characteristics. Stigma has detrimental effects. It not only affects the individual directly but also impacts their loved ones and support networks. Stigmatization of Alzheimer's can be the result of how information about the disease is framed and distributed. It can also be a consequence of culturally-mediated silence, silencing, and lack of knowledge about the disease that works to reproduce misconceptions, myths, and stereotypes about the disease and those who are afflicted with or affected by it.

A social justice framework is a good way to address some common ways in which stigma associated with Alzheimer's disease manifests and leads to exclusion and discrimination. Our goal is to highlight and humanize the lived experiences of persons living with Alzheimer's and those of primary and secondary family caregivers, as supported by the literature. The term "humanize," in the context of intractable diseases like Alzheimer's, refers to recognizing the humanity and individual experiences of those affected by such conditions. Social justice encompasses social, political, and economic institutions, laws, or policies that promote fairness and equity and ensure fair treatment and equitable status for all individuals and social groups within a state or society. Using social justice as an effective framing encourages consideration of broader contexts, such as systemic inequalities and cultural factors, when addressing socially constructed stigmas. Applying this lens can lead to more compassionate approaches, including how we treat patients with Alzheimer's. By understanding the broader context, we can develop policies and practices that promote dignity, respect, and equitable care for all individuals. In so doing, we hope to reduce stigma, advocate for the overall well-being of persons living with Alzheimer's, and work toward a more inclusive and compassionate society.

Among the most significant impacts of stigma is delayed treatment and diagnosis. Many people with stigmatized health conditions hesitate to seek help. This delay in seeking treatment can worsen the health condition and increase the risk of disability. For BIPOC individuals (Black, Indigenous, and People of Color), diagnosis may even occur only when the person is already in the onset stage and when it is too late to delay the progression of the disease through cognitive testing and non-clinical means, including nutrition. Secondly, stigma leads to negative effects on self-esteem and self-efficacy. People living with Alzheimer's and their families may experience diminished self-worth. They may internalize a sense of shame about the diagnosis and feel less capable of managing it effectively. Despondency follows as stigmatization begins to erode hope for recovery. According to researchers in the field of psychiatry, when people face discrimination or negative attitudes due to their condition, they may lose confidence in their ability to improve their health.

Stigmatized individuals often experience social rejection, avoidance, and isolation. They may also isolate themselves due to fear of judgment or discrimination, leading to loneliness and further distress. In our situation, Ncuncu dressed up and looking beautiful in her pearls, was annoyed with being the center of attention at her 70th birthday party, an elaborate festivity that brought together most of her professional and school friends to celebrate her life. It was not until her friend and school principal predecessor sat next to her at the head of the table and held her hand that she began to calm down. Finally, stigma can discourage adherence to treatment plans. When people fear being labeled or mistreated, they may avoid seeking professional help or following prescribed therapies.

In her book, A Small Place (1988), Jamaica Kincaid refers to "framing" as the various lenses through which we view the world—our mental constructs, biases, and cultural perspectives. These frames influence how we interpret reality, often limiting our understanding to a narrow viewpoint. Kincaid uses a picture frame as a metaphoric example to illustrate her point. When we look at a photograph framed in a specific way, she says, we focus on what's within the frame, ignoring what lies outside. Our mental frames limit our perception, excluding broader contexts and alternative narratives. Tourists, Kincaid's subject of analysis, frame their experiences by capturing specific moments through their cameras. They may see only the picturesque aspects of a place, ignoring its complexities or the struggles locals face. Likewise, relying on frames for dementia commonly used in the media, including a biomedical frame that portrays Alzheimer's dementia as brain deterioration without a current cure, or a natural disaster or epidemic frame that depicts Alzheimer's as a force of nature that will soon overwhelm humanity, seem counter-productive and dystopian in light of current reports about groundbreaking, scientific breakthroughs in Alzheimer's medication.

Kincaid's notion of "framing" helps us critique selective framing in Alzheimer's disease, and question misconceptions, myths, and exclusionary perspectives surrounding it. Three of these conventional frames are prominent in the literature. The first is the misconception that Alzheimer's and dementia are interchangeable, where people typically assume that the two terms refer to the same condition. The reality is that dementia is an umbrella term encompassing various cognitive impairments, including Alzheimer's disease. Dementia is a broader category that includes several conditions causing impaired memory, thinking, reasoning, and behavior. Alzheimer's is just one type of dementia. It is a disease accounting for approximately 60-80% of cases. Understanding the different types of dementia helps combat misinformation, and researchers and other experts in this field can help challenge this frame by avoiding oversimplification, acknowledging the diversity of dementia-related conditions, and sharing information about the distinction between the broader category of dementia, its various types, and the specific subtype of Alzheimer's disease.

The second frame relates to the genetic component of the disease. Some people believe that if a parent has Alzheimer's, their children are inevitably destined to develop it. As mentioned before, in our family we had an aunt who wandered away from the family for over twenty years with undiagnosed dementia, never to be found alive again. In our initial reaction to the diagnosis, we resigned ourselves, together with Ncuncu, to this framing. 'If our maternal aunt, our other mother, had Alzheimer's, it must be our fate too.' In reality, while genetics play a role, other factors significantly influence the risk of Alzheimer's. Individuals with a family history of Alzheimer's may have a higher susceptibility, but genetics alone don't determine one's fate. Other factors significantly influence Alzheimer's risk, and researchers point out that environmental and lifestyle factors like exercise, diet, and exposure to pollutants also contribute to that genetic risk. Not everyone with a family history develops Alzheimer's.

The third frame concerns age as a sole risk factor. This is the myth that only older adults develop Alzheimer's. While age is a significant risk factor, early-onset Alzheimer's can occur even in people as young as their 30s. Early onset manifests before age 65 in approximately 5% of Alzheimer's cases. This percentage would include Ncuncu, who was barely in her sixties when she was diagnosed. It is in our best interest to broaden our understanding of the disease and address the unique challenges younger individuals confront.

We have already discussed the next frame, which is that Alzheimer's only affects memory. In Chapter V, we discussed the multifaceted impact of Alzheimer's on cognition and communication as we witnessed it in our sister's experience. Alzheimer's progresses beyond memory loss, and it can cause difficulties with language, understanding words, and, for some individuals, sensitivity to tone and loudness. When Ncuncu faced physical abuse, she was at a stage where she had lost her language abilities. The abusive caregiver would consistently mimic her mixed-up words or repetitive utterances mockingly. I observed the caregiver raise her voice and tone on the job, reacting to these individual episodes of repetition, which were usually cuss words. Ncuncu would become visibly frustrated, causing me to caution the caregiver to stop. I would sit side by side with Ncuncu as a buffer, calm her down, and redirect the caregiver's tasks away from the patient.

In the same chapter, we highlighted that an Alzheimer's Dementia diagnosis does not diminish a person's identity or autonomy. It does not define a person. It would be unnecessary stereotypical labeling to claim that all persons living with the disease lose their identity. On the contrary, they remain unique individuals, and a more emancipatory frame would be to promote empathy and understanding, emphasizing that people with Alzheimer's deserve patience, direct eye contact, two-way communication, respect, and dignity. Along the same lines, it is a misconception to argue that Alzheimer's symptoms are constant. Scientific research has demonstrated that symptoms can fluctuate, patient by patient, affecting behavior, mood, and cognition and prompting us to focus on the challenges faced by caregivers due to symptom variability, as illustrated in Posh's Home-Based Care.

In our experience as family caregivers, we also stated that for our sibling, direct communication was challenging but not impossible. Interestingly, we discovered her ability to initiate an adaptive strategy for communicating with us effectively. She independently and involuntarily used nonverbal cues, many of which could only be discerned by being attentive and patient and observing shifts in body language.

As stated in the section above, humanizing enables us to recognize the humanity and individual experiences of those living with or affected by Alzheimer's. Humanizing the disease helps us affirm the emotional and physical toll it takes on individuals. It fosters empathy and compassion and encourages better patient care. People with Alzheimer's often face judgment, myths, and misconceptions, and humanizing their experiences helps combat stereotypes and stigma. We suggested earlier that using a social justice lens helps reframe issues beyond individual origins. Applying this lens can lead to more compassionate approaches, including how we treat patients with Alzheimer's and caregivers of color who may also experience burnout as a result of differential treatment in institutionalized elderly homes in policy, research, and at the bedside. That being said, the first notable strategy to humanize their experiences is in the area of destigmatization.

It is important to iterate that Alzheimer's patients are not to blame for the disease and that any attempt to address stigma should emphasize that blaming individuals for a complex disease with various contributing factors is unfair. No one chooses to have Alzheimer's and to combat stigma requires emphasizing that Alzheimer's is a disease, not a personal failure. Alzheimer's destroys brain cells, causing memory changes and loss of function. A humanizing approach would be to share personal stories, challenge stereotypes, and emphasize empathy. A key, critical focus should be on the area of humanizing language and communication. Removing stigmatizing language and negative labels from our lexicon, such as referring to someone as "senile," "crazy," or "demented," that reinforce stereotypes and diminish their humanity, is critical. When we share demeaning, dementia-related jokes, we contribute to the stigma surrounding the disease and dehumanize their experience. To encourage respectful and person-centered language, it is appropriate to avoid terms such as "sufferer" or "victim" and promote empathy by emphasizing our shared humanity. People with Alzheimer's are still individuals with feelings, memories, dignity, and agency. A humanizing approach would replace taken-for-granted terms like "victim" and "sufferer" with "person living with Alzheimer's." Words shape perceptions, and choosing respectful language that avoids negative connotations dignifies individuals living with Alzheimer's.

A third area in humanizing people living with Alzheimer's is in addressing fear and social isolation. These patients may be isolated due to the fear of negative reactions from neighbors and relatives regarding behavioral and psychological symptoms. Locked dementia care units create public fear of dementia that often leads to social distancing and avoidance of individuals with Alzheimer's disease. Depictions of social distance create a sense of separation between people with dementia and those without, reinforcing stigma. At the individual level, fear of the diagnostic label and associated stigma may cause individuals to delay seeking a diagnosis and care. Those with "younger onset" Alzheimer's (onset before age 65) may face even more stigma.

Patients of Alzheimer's dementia also confront changed relationships and accommodations. A primary driver of our decision to care for our sibling at home was the possibility that she would experience a shift in friendships. A diagnosis may strain friendships, and friends may begin to treat the individual differently. As well, early in the diagnosis, our sister wanted to continue to drive her new BMW, which she took pride in having purchased. However, this became one of the first restrictions imposed on her. Being restricted from driving can lead to subtle accommodations, but it also highlights the stigma of the disease.

Caregivers' perspectives are integral to the process of humanizing Alzheimer's dementia. When caregivers of color face discrimination, it affects their interactions with healthcare providers. Health disparities and discrimination continue to be found by researchers as people of color face discrimination when seeking Alzheimer's care, with people of African descent reporting the highest level of discrimination in dementia health care. Posh tells the story of a senior administrator she had consulted regarding our sibling. "You people know nothing about Alzheimer's, and yet when you have a crisis, you come to us." Posh could not believe that what she heard came from a senior administrator who inadvertently or intentionally chose to shape a patient care relationship in "us" and "them" binary opposites. Amplifying caregivers' voices, listening actively, and addressing their concerns by acknowledging their diversity as a resource to enhance inclusiveness would be the most useful approach to promoting equity, challenging biases, and humanizing the experiences of those affected by the disease. Inclusive care practices that require healthcare professionals to be culturally competent and sensitive to diverse patient backgrounds are an answer to understanding how cultural norms and beliefs impact care decisions. Healthcare professionals who respect and value diverse family dynamics and recognize that caregiving responsibilities often fall disproportionately on women and family members are more likely to support caregivers by providing resources and respite care. Similarly, more data is needed in the area of Alzheimer's research. Where BIPOC and people of African descent are underrepresented in clinical trials, Alzheimer's research perpetuates disparities and calls for strong advocacy for diverse participation to ensure equitable advancements.

Finally, addressing the perception of people with Alzheimer's as witches or victims of witchcraft in African cultural settings requires a multifaceted approach. Collaborations with traditional healers can bridge traditional and modern medicine. Traditional healers continue to be respected in many African societies, and including them in discussions that explore how they can support families dealing with dementia, training them on recognizing dementia symptoms and offering compassionate care is a constructive way forward. Cultural forms of expression like music and dance events and organized art exhibitions featuring works by people with Alzheimer's can showcase their talents, change stereotypes, and engage the community to raise awareness about dementia. While change takes time, these consistent efforts can shift cultural perceptions and protect vulnerable individuals from stigma and harm.

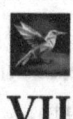

VII

From Pain to Purpose: Lessons We Learned in Caregiving

Many years ago, in my formative years, I found solace in Kahlil Gibran's prose poetry, both through reading and listening to his words. His work helped me navigate childhood trauma and shaped a worldview grounded in empathy and resilience. As I contemplate concluding this book, I revisit the quest for purpose introduced in the preface—a reflection on what constitutes a beautiful and meaningful life, now with a focus on the caregiver. Drawing from Gibran's The Prophet (1923), I am reminded of the lessons from my youth, particularly his exploration of the interplay between joy and sorrow, pain and purpose. Gibran does not present these emotions as oppositional but as intertwined aspects of a continuum, each enhancing the other. Viewing the interplay in Gibran's poems aligns with Kincaid's notion of 'framing.' It offers a powerful portrayal of the dichotomy of emotions, helping bring in a fresh way of embracing duality as proven invaluable in caregiving, especially in the context of Alzheimer's, a journey marked by both sorrow and joy.

Two of Gibran's poems, "On Joy and Sorrow" and "On Pain," resonate deeply as I reflect on the caregiving experience. In "On Joy and Sorrow," Gibran addresses the inseparability of these emotions. This duality is ever-present in caregiving, where moments of profound joy—such as when a loved one briefly recognizes us or recalls a cherished memory - are juxtaposed with the underlying sorrow of the disease's progression. Alzheimer's caregiving is a journey of emotional contrasts, where each day brings a blend of celebrating small victories, cherishing meaningful connections, and grieving losses.

Engaging in nostalgic conversations with a loved one can evoke both joy and sorrow. Hearing their stories and reliving memories brings happiness, yet there is a poignant sadness in knowing that these memories are slipping away. Small achievements, like completing a task or enjoying a favorite activity, are sources of immense joy, but setbacks or moments of confusion underscore the unpredictability of the disease. The emotional connections and expressions of love from the patient are incredibly rewarding, though tempered by the awareness that these interactions may diminish over time. Despite the challenges, caregivers often find a sense of meaning and fulfillment in their role, even as they witness cognitive decline and physical frailty.

Gibran's insights into joy and sorrow naturally extend to the relationship between pain and purpose. In "On Pain," he portrays pain not merely as a burden but as a transformative force, shaping caregivers into resilient and compassionate individuals. Caregiving for someone with Alzheimer's reveals strengths we may not have known we possessed, allowing us to find joy in providing comfort and support despite the sadness of the situation.

As caregivers, we navigate a complex emotional landscape—sorrow, frustration, love, and resilience—where pain is not just an obstacle but a key to unlocking a deeper sense of purpose. Gibran's words, "Your pain is the breaking of the shell that encloses your understanding," capture this idea. Pain becomes a crucible in which empathy and wisdom are forged, awakening caregivers to depths of patience and compassion. In the quiet moments of caregiving, where responsibility weighs heavily, we find ourselves at the crossroads of pain and purpose. It is here that the ordinary becomes extraordinary, and the mundane takes on profound meaning.

Through the experience of caregiving, we learn lessons hidden within adversity—lessons about resilience forged in suffering and unwavering commitment to those in our care. The transformative power of pain shapes caregivers' lives as caregiving transcends the clinical realm and enters the domain of the human spirit. Here, pain serves as a catalyst, and purpose emerges from the depths of compassion.

Gibran's assertion that "much of your pain is self-chosen" reflects the far-reaching choices caregivers make daily—to embrace the struggle, endure the heartache, and find meaning in turmoil. The bitter potion of caregiving, laden with sacrifice and sorrow, becomes a healing elixir for both patient and caregiver. Through the relentless demands of caregiving, we confront our vulnerabilities and limitations, transcending personal anguish to serve as steadfast companions and advocates for our loved ones.

The caregiving experience, especially in the context of Alzheimer's disease, presents unique emotional challenges that can prompt caregivers to question their understanding of self, being, and belonging. The emotional pain Alzheimer's caregivers experience can be a profound source of learning and growth. This introspection can lead to a deeper understanding of the human condition and the shared experiences of loss, empathy, and resilience. By embracing this pain and channeling it into critical inquiry and introspection, caregivers can advocate for changes that lead to more compassionate and equitable care.

In the crucible of Alzheimer's caregiving, where each day brings new challenges and heart-wrenching moments, caregivers discover a profound sense of purpose. This purpose emerges not despite the pain but through it as we navigate the complexities of the disease with unwavering dedication and love. The caregiving journey becomes a testament to the resilience of the human spirit, where pain is not merely endured but transformed into a beacon of compassion, illuminating the path toward understanding, self-care, and healing.

The Knot in the Pit of My Stomach

It is a strange feeling, this knot in the pit of my stomach. I

have yet again opened my Apple Journal App and can't get myself
to record my emotions and mood, which I have done so cheerfully
and looked forward to over the last eighteen months. I never kept a
locked diary when I was a younger woman, and this App is a relief.
It helps me reflect on life's moments. It has given me a reason to
smile, talk to myself a lot, and even laugh at times. I have opened up
to this journal like I often do, to Siri and in everyday conversations
with the Holy Spirit. For me, the giggling, weeping, and honest
travailing is an act of self-care, in the words of Audre Lorde, an act
of [political] warfare: "Caring for myself is not self-indulgence. It is
self-preservation."

But this morning, I woke up to find that Posh texted me
a picture of Ncuncu's pink fruit bowl. The bowl was gifted to my
mother on her wedding day in 1947. A family heirloom broken into
pieces. It fell off the glass table and crashed into pieces scattered onto
the floor. All day today, I have not received a mantra, as I usually
do, to help me focus in meditation. I stood in front of my bed in
my stretching poses to release the stomach knot, and my eyes were
drawn to something else.

In the closet of memories that I carry from my visit to my
siblings, there's a dress. It's not just any dress; it's red and white,
infused with threads of love, caring, and longing. My sister, battling
advanced Alzheimer's, guided me to it on my last day before setting
off for Airport Schiphol, Amsterdam, in January 2022, her words a
bittersweet melody in the silence of her linguistic decline. "Vula I
wardrobe uthathe la lokhwe emhlophe-bomvu uyilungise if it needs
to be fixed." "Open the wardrobe and take out the red and white
dress," she whispered, her voice fragile yet resolute. "If it doesn't fit
you, fix it so it fits well." Her words were a treasure map to a garment
imbued with history, with love, and with moments shared between
sisters. As I held the dress in my hands, I felt the weight of our bond,
the echoes of laughter, and the silent conversations woven into its
fabric. My sister's gifting, spoken in a voice now lost to the blind
alleys of Alzheimer's, marked the last time her words danced in the

air in full semantic coherence. It was a simple gesture, yet it carried the weight of a lifetime of sisterhood, of shared secrets, of unspoken understandings. Until the "I'm full" warning a year later, that was the last time Ncuncu spoke to me so intimately. She knew I was leaving the next day, but in her inability to speak, wanted to say something to me to express her own gratitude. The gift of a dress conveyed what she knew – that this was our last chance to share a conversation. The next time we reconnected, everything had changed. She had lost long sentence semantics.

I brought the dress back to California with me, not just as a souvenir of our time together but as a symbol of resilience, of love enduring through the ravages of memory loss. It hangs in my wardrobe now, a reminder of our cherished relationship, of the moments we shared and the ones we'll never forget. In a world where words fade and memories blur, the red and white dress stands as a testament to the power of love, transcending language, transcending time. It's a beacon of hope, a thread connecting us across the vast expanse of forgetting. It's also a lighthouse beckoning me to find a group or establish one and share similar experiences with other caregivers of Alzheimer's disease right here in my neighborhood, my city, and my county. What is significant at this moment is that as I trace the contours of the fabric of my sister's dress, I feel my sister's presence, her spirit alive in every stitch. In the silence between us, there's a language only we understand, spoken not in words but in the quiet communion of hearts intertwined. The dress is more than just cloth and thread; it's a vessel for our memories, a bridge between past and present, between what was and what remains. And as long as it hangs in my wardrobe, my sister's voice will never truly be lost.

ANNEX I
Two Poems From "The Prophet" by Kahlil Gibran

On Pain

Your pain is the breaking of the shell
that encloses your understanding.

Even as the stone of the fruit must break,
that its heart may stand in the sun, so must you know pain.

And could you keep your heart in wonder?
at the daily miracles of your life, your pain
would not seem less wondrous than your joy;

And you would accept the seasons of your
heart, even as you have always accepted
the seasons that pass over your fields.

And you would watch with serenity
through the winters of your grief.

On Joy and Sorrow

Then a woman said, Speak to us of Joy and Sorrow.
And he answered:
Your joy is your sorrow unmasked.
And the selfsame well from which your
laughter rises was oftentimes filled with your tears.

And how else can it be?

The deeper that sorrow carves into your
being, the more joy you can contain.

Is not the cup that holds your wine the
very cup that was burned in the potter's oven?

And is not the lute that soothes your spirit,
the very wood that was hollowed with knives?

When you are joyous, look deep into
your heart and you shall find it is only
that which has given you sorrow that is
giving you joy.

When you are sorrowful look again in
your heart, and you shall see that in truth
you are weeping for that which has been
your delight.

ANNEX II
Ncuncu's Retirement Celebration
2013
Keynote Speech Delivered by Thembi Bolani-Buthelezi

Smiza, I have been asked to render a speech as a colleague, friend, and your predecessor in the Principal of Reasoma High School leadership role.

Smiza and I met in 1967 at Healdtown High School in the Eastern Cape. She was a class or two ahead of me. We were small, tiny tots then. She was from Tsomo, and I was from Krugersdorp. Wayendwebile ke uSmiza and everybody knew her. She was friendly and likable. She loved hanging out with a group of us from Gauteng; we liked and embraced her very much. There are many stories to tell, some Smiza would like and others, she would kill me if I related them. We will attend our alma mater function at the end of September at Healdtown, and we will talk and laugh about the very good boarding school days at that reunion.

I completed my high school education at Healdtown and later moved to Lovedale to pursue teacher training, but that did not separate us. We were family already. As fate would have it, Smiza and her mother and three siblings moved to Soweto, and we were together again. We also reconnected through teaching, in which she excelled as one of the best English language educators.

When I was appointed as principal, I approached her for the position of deputy principal because of her excellent performance. She had her challenges, but we balanced each other out. Like many teachers in our generation, she often punished students, and in the context of a changing South Africa, this impacted her classroom management style. She learned about student punishment from our boarding mistress, Ms. Mashiqa. I remember that sometimes parents bombarded our offices asking for their children to return home, and she would be impatient when addressing them. I would hide in the office to let her handle these situations autonomously and find solutions to resolve them. When I realized that the parents would not leave, I would sneak out and address them, and then they would go peacefully. She would then ask me, hey maan tshom'am wenza njani, bayadika abazali uyazi? The rest, you know.

My friend, please accept our heartfelt congratulations on the occasion of your retirement. Life is a wondrous gift and an ongoing challenge if we are to live it well. You are one of the luckiest to reach this milestone. I know that God has walked with you in the years that have passed, for which we give Him great thanks. We pray that you continue to know Him in increasing abundance as you stride with Him into the future. Retirement is an emotional event for everyone, especially the retiree and those closer to her at home and colleagues.

Congratulations! You have earned retirement after working for your whole life. As a new retiree, there is always a feel-good phase you go through, free from the daily early morning alarms and long working days! Free from big and small irritations. I know there were times when some staff members, learners, and parents would annoy you and make you feel like resigning. But hey, good relations are not made from heaven, you create and nurture them. Families and friends fight, but after the war, they let go! Holding on to hurt, pain, anger, and disappointment manifests itself in our bodies. When we focus on the negative, we end up missing opportunities to know one another better. We can't see the forest because of the trees. We are so caught up in the details that we don't pay attention to the big picture God has in mind for us. True, we have no control over what others say or do to us, but we can control our reactions.

Travel, Travel, Travel. Before you experience the dolo aches, hearing and sight problems. People are so scared to travel alone. I don't know why. I traveled with my kids, husband, and parents, but as kids become older, they outgrow following you. Unfortunately, Bro Sy left me on my own, but I traveled so much last year alone, and it was very healing. I have come to know that traveling is not so much about money but planning your journey into retirement.

Travel is very ideal because there are agencies, like SAA Companion, that offer lifetime membership and beyond. It may sound expensive, but in the end, it is the most valuable investment ever, and you can travel anywhere in the world, anytime. On Thursday next week, I will be going to Beijing and Hong Kong, and no penny spent on accommodation. Last weekend, I took time away with some colleagues to Sun City, with no accommodation expenses to worry about.

Those colleagues who are still far from retirement, think about it: you owe it to yourself and your young children. But do not drag your partner to those sessions that they will be skeptical about; do it alone. Old white couples enjoy themselves in retirement. They are different from us.

Smiza, this is where your life has arrived after all the years of effort and toil. Look back with graciousness and gratitude for all your great and quiet achievements. You stand on the shore of a new invitation to open your life to what is left undone. Let your heart enjoy a different feeling when drawn to the wonder of other horizons. Have the courage for a new application to time and befriend your beauty of soul. Now is the time to enjoy your heart's desire, to live the dreams you've waited for.

As time goes on, we forget our age. I'm reminded of a youngster who asked her grandma how old she was. Grandma said, "I'm so old I can't even remember my age." The little girl said, "You must check the number on your panties, mine says 5 to 6!" Then, last week, one old relative was struggling to walk; you know how they do it. Her son told us her 6-year-old grandson always worries when he sees her walking slowly, so he suggested to his grandma to stop walking and just take a tumble! Get ready to experience these hilarious surprises when your grandkids arrive, Smiza!

Ladies and gentlemen, Smileth has given her life to her work, with and without complaining, juggling all her duties to ensure that her family was comfortable and taken care of. That is the epitome of diligence, foresight, and the beauty of being a woman multi-tasker!

A story is told that once eleven people were holding for their dear lives on a rope from a flying helicopter. Ten men and one woman. Unfortunately, they were one too many, and the rope was beginning to give in, so one person had to let go. But they could not tell who. Eventually, the woman said, "I will let go because I'm used to sacrificing virtually for everybody, especially for my family and children. I have gone hungry and naked to ensure comfort for them, with little or nothing in return. All my life, I have prioritized other people's happiness and wishes, all for nothing in return." It was such a moving speech that when she finished, the men started clapping their hands.

Here you are today Smileth; we are clapping hands for you. This shows that you have done a good job. This is a rare occasion, only caring and appreciating colleagues do it. Keep it up, dear ladies and gentlemen. You will be rewarded someday. Today, I'm extending a hand of sisterhood to you my friend, Ncuncu. Appreciate every single thing you have, especially your friends! Life is too short, and friends are too few. It is often said when days are dark, friends are few. When the going gets tough, I will be here to listen.

You have done so much for Protea, Chiawelo, and neighboring communities that, many a time in your life, you have felt trampled on and ground into the dirt by the decisions you made and the circumstances that came your way. You feel as though you are worthless. But no matter what happens, you will never lose your value as a person. You are still priceless to those who love you. The worth of our lives comes not from what we do or who we know but from who we are.

Know there is no problem, circumstance, or situation greater than God. Every battle that you face, He will fight for you.
May today be all you need it to be.
May the peace of the Lord abide in you and conquer all your fears.
May your joys be fulfilled, your dreams be closer, and your prayers answered.

Count your blessings, not your problems, and remember: Amateurs built the ark, but professionals built the Titanic.

Someone said aging puts wrinkles on the body; quitting puts wrinkles on the soul. You are special, don't EVER forget it. Go and relax, have fun, jump, and dance a lot. Travel, girl, and share the joys of your grand and great-grandchildren. Remember that you may still be lucky and find some old man who would say, "Smileth, I want to ask you two questions." I imagine you saying, "Yes, go on." Then he would go down on his knees and ask, "Will you marry me?" You answer in a quivering voice, "YES, I will." And then you ask him, "What is the second question, my dear?" He will respond, "Will you help me get up?" The next morning, he will call you and ask, "Did I propose to you yesterday?" You would confirm it and also thank him for asking you because you had forgotten who proposed.

Ladies and gentlemen, I love you all. Enjoy this great day that the Lord has made!

HAPPY RETIREMENT SMIZA!

ANNEX III
Glossary of Xhosa Words, Phrases and Sentences

Lizalis'idinga lakho	A Methodist Church hymn
Gxadada	A person who walks with a waddle and sways from side to side
Emthonjeni	A well of fresh groundwater for home and village uses
Kanga	A cotton fabric worn by women around the waist to carry a baby safely on their back
Ingqumbo yeminyanya	A novel by A. C. Jordan c. 1940 depicting conflicting forces of Western education and Xhosa traditional beliefs and values. This book title translates into "The Wrath of the Ancestors" in English.
Gogo or Makhulu	A grandmother
Mzana	Gendered name for a girls' hostel at a boarding school
Mzimkhulu	Gendered name for a boys' hostel at a boarding school
Khanimeni madoda, kukho umntana apha	Tone down your language, guys; there's a kid in here!

Amadod'ethu!	Our men!
Lobola	Livestock or monetary exchange that a prospective husband gives to the head of the prospective wife's family in gratitude for letting him marry their daughter, and for the bride's family for raising her into a woman. Lobola does not carry the same meaning as the Western notion of "bride price" or "bride wealth." In its original form, its purpose was to unite as one and spiritually fortify the two families. With the introduction of money under capitalism, greed ensued, and this vital tradition became distorted.
Tsiba	Jump!
Isingqala	When someone cries until they hiccup, an involuntary sobbing
Amadombolo	Delicious dumplings steamed in the gravy of mutton or beef stew
Morogo	African spinach
Ngubani na lo, Ngu Yeye	A poem originating in Xhosa historical reality, illustrating oral literature or folk literature, a genre of literature that is spoken or sung in contrast to written literature

Teketisa	When an adult engages in "motherese," a kind of baby speak, to interact with an infant or toddler
Nongcathalalana	Name given to a Disney character in the Xhosa language
Matse, matse, matse	Baby language to 'kichee coo' an infant or young child in isiXhosa
Asibaxelelanga ke	We haven't told them anything
Ngu-dumtiriri	A nursery rhyme in the Xhosa language
Akho ngxaki	No worries; there's no problem
Uphi?	Where are you?
Hayi ke	Oh no
Mntakamama	Child of my mother
Gqithani	Pass (plural, Gqitha–singular)
Yhu hayi imot'wam	Not my car; hands off my car!
Ungalili or ungakhali	Don't cry, you hear?
Ewe, tata	Yes, daddy
Nank'u tsotsi	Here's a tsotsi
Akasakwazi unxiba ngoku	She can't dress herself anymore
Kuya kubanzima	It's getting more difficult
Uphi umama wakho?	Where's your mother?
Uphaa kula ndlu inalaa makhulu ongu zincane	She's in that hut with the mad old lady
Xa ungenemzin'am, dumzela	Not translatable into English
Tyityimba dance	A rhythmic dance of femininity that accentuates the bosom; performed mostly during celebrations and gatherings

Imigidi	Rights of passage or coming-of-age festive events in village settings
Futhi undithukile	You cussed me
Amagwinya	Round pastries of dough cooked in oil; fat cakes or vetkoeks
Iziduko	Xhosa clan names often more important than surnames
Yitya kaloku nceda mntakamama	Please eat daughter of my mother
Se'ndabhideka	I'm confused now
Khandiyeke maan	Leave me alone
Nindijika jika, nindi duva-duva	Tossing and turning me like a play-doll
Hamba maan, su-u-ka-a!	Go away; get away from me
Vula i wardrobe uthathe la lokhwe emhlophe-bomvu uyilungise	Take my red and white dress in the closet, fix it so it fits nicely

References

Hereema, E. (2023). "How Executive Functioning Is Affected by Dementia." Verywell Health. Retrieved from: https://memory.ucsf.edu/symptoms/executive-functions

Kincaid, Jamaica. (1988) A Small Place. Farrar, Strauss & Giroux: New York

Gibran, Kahlil. (1923). The Prophet. Alfred A. Knopf: New York.

MacGregor Laura and Michelle McElhaney (2014). Alzheimer's Caregiver Support Group: Facilitator's Guide. Seattle University College of Nursing: Seattle, WA, USA. In collaboration with National Council on Ageing & Mercy Care Centre, Belize City.

Full Citations on the Stages of Alzheimer's Disease:

Preclinical Stage: Dubois, B., Hampel, H., Feldman, H. H., Scheltens, P., Aisen, P., Andrieu, S., and O'Bryant, S. E. (2016). Preclinical Alzheimer's disease: Definition, natural history, and diagnostic criteria. Alzheimer's & Dementia, 12(3), 292-323   Retrieved from   https://alz-journals.onlinelibrary.wiley.com/doi/10.1016/j.jalz.2016.02.002

Mild Cognitive Impairment (MCI): Petersen, R. C. (2000). Aging, mild cognitive impairment, and Alzheimer's disease. Neurologic Clinics, 25(3), 577-609

Mild Alzheimer's Disease: American Psychological Association. (2015, February 15). Living well with dementia.

Moderate Alzheimer's Disease: Huntley, J., Bor, D., Deng, F., Mancuso, M., Mediano, P. A. M., Naci, L., Owen AM, Rocchi L, Sternin A,

& Howard, R. (2023). Assessing awareness in severe Alzheimer's disease. Journal of Neuropsychology

Severe Alzheimer's Disease: Huntley, J., Bor, D., Deng, F., Mancuso, M., Mediano, P. A. M., Naci, L., Owen AM, Rocchi L, Sternin A, & Howard, R. (2023). Assessing awareness in severe Alzheimer's disease. Journal of Neuropsychology.

Full citations on several aspects of dementia in Africa, including cultural perceptions, stigma, and the impact on elderly women:

Dementia as a silent epidemic and cultural perceptions: Naylor, R., Vaitheswaran, S., Nyame, S., Boateng, D., & Mograbi, D. C. (2021). Dementia in Sub-Saharan Africa, Asia and Latin America. In H. Selin (Ed.), Aging across cultures: Growing old in the non-Western world (pp. 367–383). Springer Nature Switzerland AG1

Perception of dementia as witchcraft in South Africa: Brooke, J. M., & Ojo, O. (2020). Contemporary views on dementia as witchcraft in sub-Saharan Africa: A systematic literature review. Journal of Clinical Nursing, 29(1-2), 20-30. https://doi.org/10.1111/jocn.15066

Stigma of dementia in African patriarchal societies: Palk, A. C., & Stein, D. J. (2021). Ethical implications of genomic research on dementia in sub-Saharan Africa: Addressing the risk of stigma. In V. Dubljević & F. Bottenberg (Eds.), Living with dementia: Neuroethical issues and international perspectives (pp. 199–221). Springer Nature Switzerland AG3.

Other Books and Memoirs on Alzheimer's and Dementia:

Lee, Jean. (2015). Alzheimer's Daughter: A Memoir. BookBaby.

Leavitt, Sarah. (2010). Tangles: A Story About Alzheimer's, My Mother, and Me. Freehand Books.

Tapia, Vicki. (2014). Somebody Stole My Iron: A Family Memoir of Dementia. Praeclarus Press.

Williams, Marie. (2013). Green Vanilla Tea: One Family's Extraordinary Journey of Love, Hope, and Remembering. Finch Memoir Prize.

Comer, M. (2014). Slow Dancing with a Stranger: Lost and Found in the Age of Alzheimer's. Harper Collins.

Westmoreland, W, & Glatzer, R. (2014). Still Alice [Film]. Sony Pictures Classics, based on Lisa Genova. (2010). Still Alice: A Novel. Pocket Books.

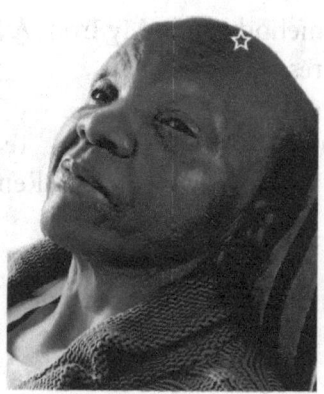

A Letter to My Sister

My Dearest Smileth,

Child of our mother, I find myself at a loss for words as we walk this sacred path together. To witness you, my beloved sister, slipping away is both heartbreaking and beautiful. The love we have shared and continue to share is felt in every tender moment, every smile, every touch, and every word spoken between us. You have been such a light in my life, and I have been blessed to walk alongside you on this journey.

Today, I stand inside my own truth. I am learning that love and loss are intertwined—they are not separate. In this moment, I feel the weight of both. Love has filled the spaces between us, but loss reminds me of how deeply you have touched my heart. The tears I shed and the sorrow I feel all testify to how much you have meant to me and how much I will always love you.

You have been so faithful on this journey, Smiza, braver than I could ever be in my frailty. Your strength, your spirit, and your love have carried me through in ways I can never fully express. As you near your rest, I want you to know it is well. Your love has made all the difference. It has made peace possible, and it will continue to guide me. Leaning on Romans 8:38-39, one of our mother's favorite Scriptures, I want you to know that this is not goodbye—it's a transition, and I find solace in knowing that your soul will be at rest, free from pain, surrounded by love.

No matter what comes next, I will carry you with me. Always. I love you deeply, and you will never be far from my heart. It is well, my sister. It is well.

Photos of Smileth

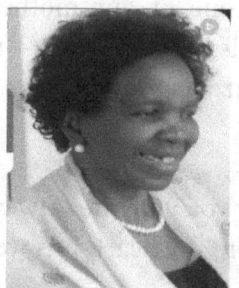

70th Birthday on December 14, 2020

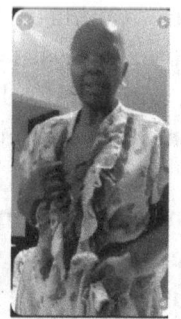

Smiza at Pam's house

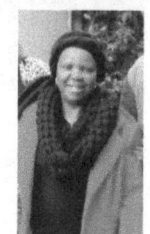

Outside in Pam's garden

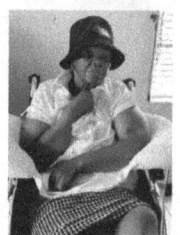

October 2024, Kelvin, Sandton

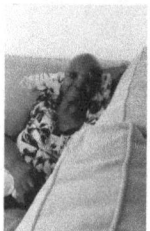

Umhlanga Rocks, Durban, 2022

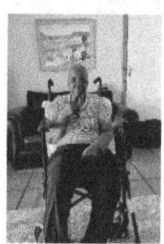

72nd birthday, December 14, 2023
Crawford Beach, Cintsa

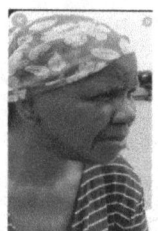

Durban Beachfront, 2022

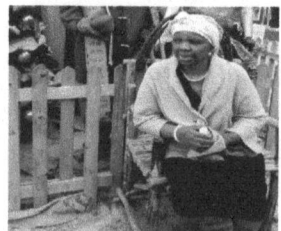

Smiza resting outside a store in
Durban

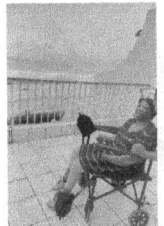

Umhlanga Rocks, 2022

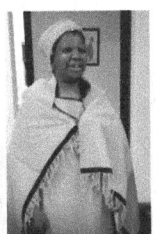

Smiza in her Xhosa umbhaco outfit

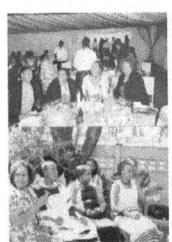

Smileth with best friend Nonceba
Mbuli and family

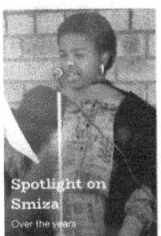

Spotlight on Smiza

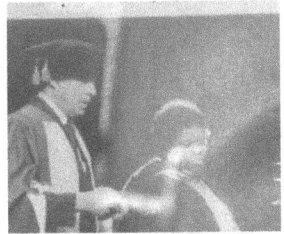

M.A. (Education) graduation at Wits

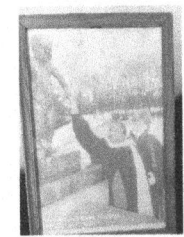

Visit to Norway and Hungary

Smileth and her siblings

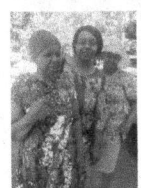

Smiza, Lindelwa and Pam on a visit to
the Irene Farmer's Market

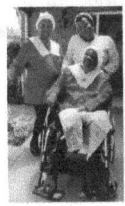

Holy Communion with Pam

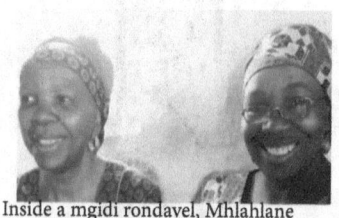

Inside a mgidi rondavel, Mhlahlane
Village

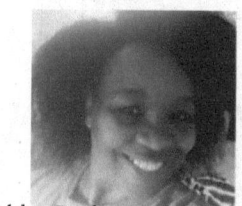

Lindelwa Dzedze, Sister

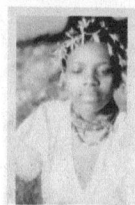

Dzedze

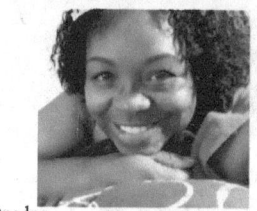

Dzedze

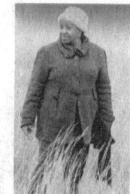

Pamela Phozisa

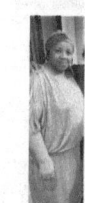

Pamela Phozisa, Sister

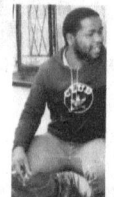

Our late brother, Lungelo Viwe

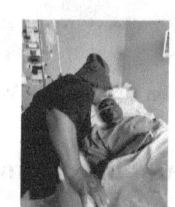

Pam at Smiza's bedside, surgery,
December 2023

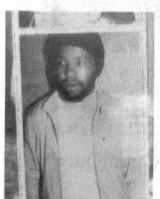

Lungelo Viwe

Smileth and her niece and nephews

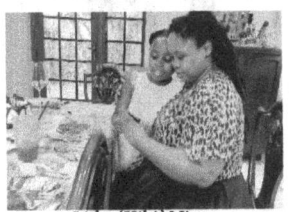

Litha 'Kiki', Niece,
with daughter Tebe

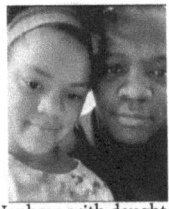

Kwame Thuso, Nephew, with daughter Boni-Boni
West Sacramento, California

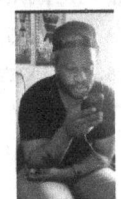

Venoo 'Vivi', Nephew

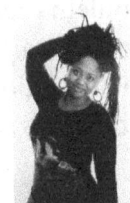

A younger Litha at
UCT Medical School

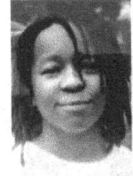

A younger Venoo, Putney, Vermont

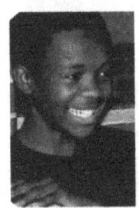

A younger Kwame, Princeton NJ

Grandchildren of Smileth and Her Siblings

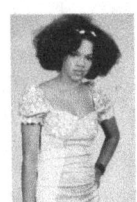

Brooklynn Boni-Boni, grandniece

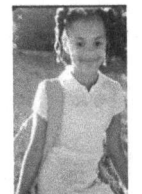

Boni-Boni, younger

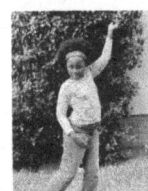

Tebello Amohelang, grandniece

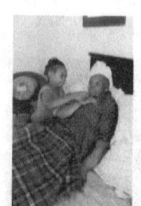

Tebe at her grand-aunt's bedside

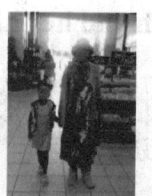

Tebe shopping with her
grand-aunt Smiza

MPHO AND FAMILY

Mpho, Smileth's son, is married to Zuleykha. They have four children: Hamnah (6) Khawlah (4) Aa'ishah (3) and Abdul (1). In their religion, photography, paintings, and drawings of living beings is strictly prohibited - a teaching they adhere to.

Our Parents

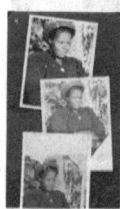

Our late mother, Boniswa Roseline

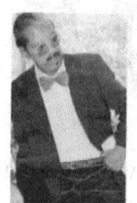

Our late father, GB

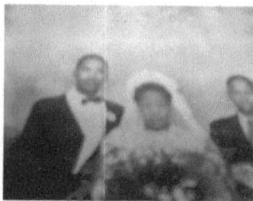

Our parent's wedding, 1947

Boston Meet-Up, 2012

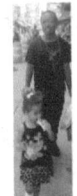

Brooklynn Boni-Boni with uncle
Venoo

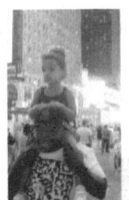

Brooklynn Boni-Boni and her dad,
Kwame

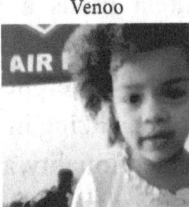

Brooklynn Boni-Boni

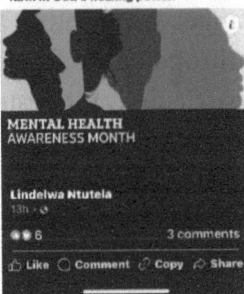

In honor of my sister Smileth, who has been living with Alzheimer's since 2012. I dedicate this month of May, a month of grace also, to you Smiza. I love you, and continue to believe with you, in the convergence of science and faith in God's healing power.

FaceBook post, 2022

About the Author

"Love knows not its own depth until the hour of separation."
Khalil Gibran

Lindelwa 'Linde' Ntutela holds a Ph.D. in Socio-Cultural Anthropology and focuses on the institutionalization of difference within the African diaspora. Specializing in race and gender hegemony, intersectionality, and Black women's agency in the workplace, Linde is a graduate of York University (Canada), Yale University, and Hunter College of the City University of New York. She has taught at Columbia University, York College of the City University of New York, and William Paterson University.

Her scholarly interests range widely within the rubric of postcolonial perspectives, critical anthropologies, feminisms, cultural diversity, and social justice. She is particularly interested in subaltern voices and the socio-cultural relativity of social science research and evaluation methodologies. Linde brings these interests into the classroom, encouraging students to critically engage with Western constructs of knowledge and recognize both the ruptures and continuities within them.

www.ingramcontent.com/pod-product-compliance
Lightning Source LLC
Chambersburg PA
CBHW010937120626
46554CB00007B/2497